MRSA

MRSA

EDITED BY

JOHN A. WEIGELT, M.D.

MEDICAL COLLEGE OF WISCONSIN
DIVISION OF TRAUMA AND CRITICAL CARE
DEPARTMENT OF SURGERY
MILWAUKEE, WISCONSIN, USA

informa

healthcare

New York   London

Informa Healthcare USA, Inc.
52 Vanderbilt Avenue
New York, NY 10017

No claim to original U.S. Government works
Printed in Canada on acid-free paper
10 9 8 7 6 5 4 3 2 1

International Standard Book Number-10: 1-4200-4549-0 (Softcover)
International Standard Book Number-13: 978-1-4200-4549-9 (Softcover)

This book contains information obtained from authentic and highly regarded sources. Reprinted material is quoted with permission, and sources are indicated. A wide variety of references are listed. Reasonable efforts have been made to publish reliable data and information, but the author and the publisher cannot assume responsibility for the validity of all materials or for the consequence of their use.

Library of Congress Cataloging-in-Publication Data

MRSA / edited by John A. Weigelt.
  p. ; cm.
  Includes bibliographical references and index.
  ISBN-13: 978-1-4200-4549-9 (alk. paper)
  ISBN-10: 1-4200-4549-0 (alk. paper)
  1. Staphylococcus aureus infections--Chemotherapy 2. Methicillin resistance. I. Weigelt, John A. II. Title: Methicillin-resistant staphylococcus aureus.
  [DNLM: 1. Staphylococcal Infections--prevention & control. 2. Methicillin Resistance. 3. Staphylococcus aureus--drug effects. WC 250 M9385 2007]
  QR201.S68M77 2007
  616.9'297061--dc22
                                                          2006051465

Visit the Informa Web site at
www.informa.com

and the Informa Healthcare Web site at
www.informahealthcare.com

Preface

Staphylococcus aureus continues to be a compelling subject. This bacterium has been extraordinary in reinventing itself and keeping one step ahead of therapeutic advances. First, *S. aureus* left penicillin in its wake, and now methicillin and the cephalosporins are becoming impotent antibiotics. Even vancomycin has been challenged in a number of ways as *S. aureus* continues to evolve its genetic make-up.

In writing about *S. aureus* infection assessment and management, the chapter authors of this volume were faced with a constantly evolving medical science. All of the authors are experts with a passion for providing optimal care to patients with *S. aureus* infections. We have tried our best to discuss *S. aureus* from a clinical perspective and to define how methicillin-resistant *S. aureus* or MRSA has altered our opinions of gram-positive infections.

The chapters deal with separate but often overlapping topics related to the diagnosis and management of MRSA infections. We start with a historical note and work our way through the differentiation of community-acquired and hospital-acquired MRSA infections. Understanding the epidemiology of this bacterium as well as new treatment options were our major goals. These final chapters constitute our best understanding of this bacterium today, and the authors have done an outstanding job. Naturally *S. aureus* will continue to evolve and management options will need to be modified accordingly.

I sincerely thank all the authors who were kind enough to understand that this book needed to be completed expediently so that we could get current information quickly into the hands of clinicians. This is important since clinicians all around the world are facing an everchanging challenge from MRSA. This challenge involves not only the bacterium itself but also the type of disease that it causes. This book provides healthcare providers with current information on new treatment options as well as recommendations for prevention. While all the answers are not yet available, this book offers some assistance to clinicians.

John A. Weigelt

Contents

Contributors

David G. Armstrong The Center for Lower Extremity Ambulatory Research (CLEAR), Dr. William M. Scholl College of Podiatric Medicine, Rosalind Franklin University of Medicine and Science, Chicago, Illinois, U.S.A.

Nicholas J. Bevilacqua The Center for Lower Extremity Ambulatory Research (CLEAR), Dr. William M. Scholl College of Podiatric Medicine, Rosalind Franklin University of Medicine and Science, Chicago, Illinois, U.S.A.

Karen J. Brasel Department of Surgery, Medical College of Wisconsin, Milwaukee, Wisconsin, U.S.A.

Melissa Brunsvold Department of Surgery, University of Michigan Medical System, Ann Arbor, Michigan, U.S.A.

Kent Crossley Department of Medicine, Veterans Affairs Medical Center and the University of Minnesota Medical School, Minneapolis, Minnesota, U.S.A.

Charles E. Edmiston, Jr. Department of Surgery, Medical College of Wisconsin, Milwaukee, Wisconsin, U.S.A.

Barry C. Fox Department of Medicine, University of Wisconsin Medical School and University of Wisconsin Hospital and Clinics, and the William S. Middleton Veterans Affairs Medical Center, Madison, Wisconsin, U.S.A.

Kamal M. F. Itani Department of Surgery, Boston Veterans Affairs Health Care System, Boston University, Boston, Massachusetts, U.S.A.

Anna P. Lam Division of Pulmonary and Critical Care Medicine, Feinberg School of Medicine, Northwestern University, Chicago, Illinois, U.S.A.

Thomas P. Lodise, Jr. Department of Pharmacy Practice, Albany College of Pharmacy, Albany, New York, U.S.A.

Linda M. McKinley Department of Infection Control, the William S. Middleton Veterans Affairs Medical Center, Madison, Wisconsin, U.S.A.

Peggy S. McKinnon Department of Pharmacy, Clinical Research and Infectious Diseases, Barnes-Jewish Hospital, St. Louis, Missouri, U.S.A.

Lena M. Napolitano Department of Surgery, University of Michigan Medical System, Ann Arbor, Michigan, U.S.A.

R. Lawrence Reed Surgical Intensive Care Unit, Edward Hines, Jr. Veterans Affairs Hospital and Department of Surgery, Loyola University Medical Center, Maywood, Illinois, U.S.A.

Lee C. Rogers The Center for Lower Extremity Ambulatory Research (CLEAR), Dr. William M. Scholl College of Podiatric Medicine, Rosalind Franklin University of Medicine and Science, Chicago, Illinois, U.S.A.

Nasia Safdar Department of Medicine, University of Wisconsin Medical School and University of Wisconsin Hospital and Clinics, and the William S. Middleton Veterans Affairs Medical Center, Madison, Wisconsin, U.S.A.

Renae E. Stafford Department of Surgery, University of North Carolina, Chapel Hill, North Carolina, U.S.A.

Dennis Stevens Infectious Diseases Section, Veterans Affairs Medical Center, Boise, Idaho, and Department of Medicine, University of Washington, Seattle, Washington, U.S.A.

John A. Weigelt Department of Surgery, Medical College of Wisconsin, Milwaukee, Wisconsin, U.S.A.

Richard G. Wunderink Division of Pulmonary and Critical Care Medicine, Feinberg School of Medicine, Northwestern University, Chicago, Illinois, U.S.A.

Overview of *Staphylococcus aureus* in Medicine

Kent Crossley
Department of Medicine, Veterans Affairs Medical Center and the University of Minnesota Medical School, Minneapolis, Minnesota, U.S.A.

INTRODUCTION

Staphylococcus aureus has been a major cause of infections in humans for as long as we have historical records. Pathological changes consistent with staphylococcal osteomyelitis are known from Egyptian mummies and other remains of similar antiquity. Along with several other organisms (e.g., group A β-hemolytic streptococci and *Mycobacterium tuberculosis*), this organism is uniquely equipped with virulence factors and defense mechanisms that enable it to cause rapidly progressive fatal infections in normal individuals.

In striking contrast to bacteria such as *S. aureus* and Group A β-streptococci, many of the organisms that cause healthcare-associated infections lack well-developed virulence factors and are only able to cause infection because of the absence of normal defenses in the compromised host. Gram-negative bacteria (e.g., *Pseudomonas* or *Serratia*) and fungi (*Candida* or *Aspergillus* species) rarely cause serious infection in normal hosts.

COMMUNITY- AND HOSPITAL-ASSOCIATED INFECTION

Staphylococcus aureus is a major cause of both healthcare- and community-acquired infections. It is perhaps the single most common cause of healthcare-associated infection throughout the world (1). Although data are less extensive about community-acquired infection, it is a frequent cause of skin and soft tissue infection, bacteremia, and endocarditis. *Staphylococcus aureus*, almost uniquely among common pathogens, also has an astonishing history of changing clinical manifestations and epidemiologic behavior. The sudden appearance of toxic shock syndrome (TSS) and the continuing parallel evolution of antibiotic resistance and virulence are two examples.

Staphylococci are recognized as common causes of osteomyelitis, skin and soft tissue infections, and bacteremia in normal hosts. Although there are few recent surveys of the causes of community-associated bacteremia, *S. aureus* is a frequent isolate and one that is also associated with significant morbidity and mortality (2,3). Although most *S. aureus* infections are minor episodes of cellulitis or cutaneous abscesses, serious infections associated with severe systemic toxicity and an abrupt death are not infrequent. Most experienced physicians remember one or more normal young patients who developed bacteremia and endocarditis from a trivial localized infection or who may have developed staphylococcal pneumonia and died in a few days. Rapidly progressive and often fatal infection has recently been seen in normal young individuals infected with community-acquired methicillin-resistant *S. aureus* (MRSA) infections caused by isolates that contain the Panton–Valentine leukocidin (PVL) (4).

Staphylococcal infection in hospitalized patients has been of major concern for well over a century. Even before the organism was named in the 1880s, clusters of gram-positive cocci had been recognized as the usual cause of suppuration in infected wounds. The gradual introduction of components of "aseptic technique" helped to reduce the frequency of these postoperative infections. The advent of the sulfonamides and penicillins was followed by dramatic reduction in the frequency of these infections. By the 1950s, however, prior to the introduction of the semisynthetic penicillins (e.g., methicillin or oxacillin), penicillin-resistant staphylococci had become a major problem in U.S. hospitals. The introduction of vancomycin and the anti-staphylococcal penicillins again brought these infections under control until the arrival of MRSA. Much of the current attention to MRSA is reminiscent of the publicity and anxiety associated with staphylococcal infections in the 1950s.

Thus, long before recognition of MRSA as a hospital-associated pathogen, *S. aureus* had been a major problem in healthcare. Examination of National Nosocomial Infection Survey data from the 1980s indicates that *S. aureus* was always one of the most frequent pathogens recovered in hospitals and that it was the most common cause of surgical wound infection (5). Although a relatively uncommon isolate from the urine, *S. aureus* was also recognized as a frequent cause of hospital-associated pneumonia, vascular catheter-associated infection, abscesses, other skin and soft tissue infection, and bacteremia.

METHICILLIN-RESISTANT *STAPHYLOCOCCUS AUREUS*

MRSA was first recognized in the United States in an outbreak reported at Boston City Hospital in the late 1960s (6). These resistant staphylococci were already well established in major European hospitals by that time. For unclear reasons, there were relatively few cases of infection with this organism in the United States until the middle of the following decade. By 1975, outbreaks of MRSA were being reported with regularity from teaching hospitals and especially from hospitals and from units that cared for patients who had been burned (7). Since that time, the frequency of MRSA in hospitalized patients in the United States has continued to grow. Although rates increased, geographic and institutional variation was also recognized. Nonetheless, an overall inexorable progressive increase in the frequency of this organism in hospitals and in other healthcare facilities (such as nursing homes) has occurred.

Although rarely discussed, it is fascinating that MRSA has not replaced more susceptible *S. aureus* as a pathogen (8). Healthcare institutions have continued to have a baseline number of *S. aureus* hospital-associated infections caused by methicillin-sensitive strains. Infections caused by MRSA are additive to this baseline. Thus, an institution which had 15% of its nosocomial infections caused by *S. aureus* prior to

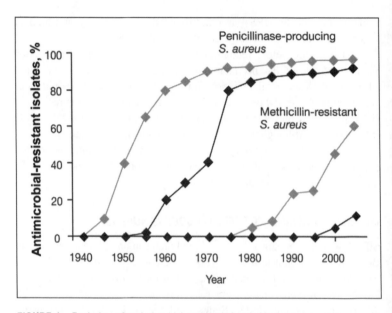

FIGURE 1 Evolution of antimicrobial-resistant *Staphylococcus aureus* as a cause of nosocomial and, then, community-acquired infections. *Key*: *Black squares*, nosocomial infection; *gray squares*, community-acquired infection.

encountering problems with MRSA might, in the following year, have 15% of nosocomial infections caused by sensitive *S. aureus* and an additional 15% caused by MRSA (Fig. 1) (1). This is a major reason that staphylococci are now of so much concern in healthcare. They are simply more frequent than most other causes of nosocomial infection. It is reported that nearly 1% of patients discharged from U.S. hospitals in 2000 and 2001 had *S. aureus* infection. These patients were found to have three times the length of hospitalization, three times the total hospital charges, and five times the risk of in-hospital death when compared with inpatients without staphylococcal infection (9).

When staphylococci resistant to penicillin were first seen in the 1950s, they were isolated from patients in hospitals. However, in a relatively few years, these organisms began to replace penicillin-susceptible staphylococci in community-associated infections. A similar process has recently happened with MRSA. Although these isolates were first seen in large acute care hospitals, over the last 10 years they have become frequent isolates from typical community-acquired staphylococcal infections. Thus, a patient presenting to an emergency room or urgent care with a carbuncle or infected laceration in 2007 may well have an MRSA isolated even though the patient has not had recent contact with a healthcare facility.

This recent movement of MRSA into the community differs in a major way when compared with the spread of penicillin-resistant staphylococci some 50 years ago. The hospital-associated MRSA have not simply "migrated" into the community. The community-associated MRSA (CA-MRSA) are distinct in a variety of ways from the isolates recovered in hospitals. Although the reasons for this are complex, and not entirely understood, it would appear that the genetic determinants of methicillin resistance have been grafted into strains of *S. aureus* that are "epidemiologically virulent." These are organisms that have the necessary virulence factors to be able to cause serious acute infections in normal individuals. They also typically carry other genetic information that allows them to effectively spread between individuals and be effective colonizers. With the addition of the genetic determinant of methicillin resistance (called MecA and carried by a plasmid-like element called the *Staphylococcus* cassette chromosome), strains that are epidemiologically and clinically virulent have become much more problematic for therapy. These CA-MRSA have also been associated with a number of outbreaks of infections in hospitals.

EPIDEMIOLOGY OF STAPHYLOCOCCAL INFECTION

Key to understanding how staphylococcal infections develop is an appreciation of the habits of this organism (10). Soon after birth, many neonates become colonized in the anterior nares with *S. aureus*. In adults, 20% to 45% of normal individuals will carry this organism in their anterior nares. Although not understood, it is well recognized that people who frequently use needles, whether for insulin administration, desensitization to allergens, or illicit recreational drug administration, have higher carrier rates than other individuals.

The carrier state is well documented to be significantly associated with the development of infections when an injury or skin break occurs. A patient known to be nasally colonized with *S. aureus* has a significantly higher risk of developing staphylococcal wound infection after a surgical procedure than someone who is not colonized (11). It is also clear that patients who develop bacteremia with *S. aureus* are usually nasally colonized with the same strain that is recovered from the blood (12). Carriage is a complex topic and it has been extensively studied. Some individuals appear to be chronically colonized; others are only intermittent carriers. Those individuals who are chronically colonized ("persistent carriers") are at highest risk for development of infection following a surgical procedure. In addition to nasal colonization, staphylococci also colonize the peritoneum as well as cutaneous wounds, especially in individuals who are nasal carriers. Although the throat is commonly colonized, the importance of this is not well understood. Carriage is not just a human phenomenon. Household pets may also carry *S. aureus* and have played an important role in some family outbreaks of *S. aureus* disease.

Many individuals who work in hospitals may be nasally colonized. The frequency varies with the extent and type of patient contact. These healthcare workers often carry the organisms on their fingertips; this is believed to be a consequence of nasal colonization and of hand contamination from other patients and the inanimate environment. Passing staphylococci between patients on the hands of healthcare workers is the most frequent way in which these organisms are spread within the healthcare environment. Prevention of these infections requires careful hand washing or sanitization on the part of healthcare workers.

Staphylococcus aureus, like most bacteria, has a variety of structural and enzymatic components that may function in different ways depending on the environment. This enables optimal efficiency for the organism. When there are no antibiotics in the environment, the bacteria has no need to expend energy to maintain antibiotic resistance. The same principle applies to staphylococci as colonizers. Organisms present in the nose are in a semidormant metabolic state. However, once staphylococci reach a site such as a new wound, the organisms have the ability to elaborate a variety of enzymes and toxins that allow them to invade tissues. These same virulence factors are toxic to polymorphonuclear leukocytes and other cells of host defense. Many isolates of *S. aureus* can also elaborate a capsule that, as one of its functions, allows the organism to avoid phagocytosis. Once taken up by human leukocytes, staphylococci are often able to survive for extended periods of time, and revert to a semidormant state.

CLINICAL INFECTIONS

Skin and Soft Tissue

Staphylococcus aureus may infect any organ or tissue of the body. Infections of the skin, soft tissue, and bone are the most frequent. These infections may range from a localized abscess to more generalized infections such as cellulitis or impetigo. Staphylococcal osteomyelitis is typically the result of a bacteremia in young children, but in older individuals it is related to an adjacent site of infection. Septic bursitis is another common staphylococcal infection. This often involves the olecranon bursa and is almost always caused by *S. aureus*. *Staphylococcus aureus* is also a frequent cause of vascular catheter-associated infection, postoperative wound infection, and other infections that are uniquely associated with healthcare.

Although any type of *S. aureus* infection can be associated with development of TSS, at the present time, most patients with this illness have infections involving skin and soft tissue. Originally reported as a complication of tampon use in women who had vaginal colonization with *S. aureus*, TSS is now seen only infrequently. Patients presenting with weakness, postural hypotension, a diffuse pale macular rash, conjunctival injection, and evidence of a localized staphylococcal infection may have TSS.

Bacteremia and Endocarditis

Staphylococcus aureus accounts for between 15% and 25% of episodes of bacteremia in large-scale studies (2). In individuals who develop their infection in the community, vascular insufficiency and insulin-dependent diabetes are associated with an increased frequency of staphylococcal bacteremia. In hospitalized patients, monitoring devices or vascular catheters are often implicated as the source. Mortality in patients with *S. aureus* bacteremia remains between 5% and 30% even with effective antibiotic therapy. Patients with no obvious portal of entry, elderly individuals, and those with serious underlying diseases are at particular risk for death. Identification and management of the source of bacteremia, including early catheter removal, is imperative.

Staphylococcus aureus is the most frequent cause of acute bacterial endocarditis. It may be acquired in the hospital or community. Most cases are a consequence of an infection acquired as a result of a healthcare intervention (13). *Staphylococcus aureus* is capable of causing lethal infection in individuals who do not have pre-existing valvular disease. In general, these infections are on the left side of the heart and usually require valve replacement for cure. The use of blood cultures and cardiac ultrasound are usual routes for identifying staphylococcal cardiac infection. Sophisticated clinically-derived algorithms are often used to differentiate between uncomplicated bacteremia and the presence of endocarditis (14).

Untreated *S. aureus* bacteremia may be associated with metastatic infection. Patients may develop abscesses involving tissue such as the liver, spleen, or even muscle secondary to bacteremia. Persisting clinical evidence of infections should lead to a methodical search for additional loci of staphylococcal infection in patients who are, or have been, bacteremic.

Pneumonia

Staphylococcus aureus pneumonia was recognized infrequently in the past and was primarily seen as a complication of influenza. Many of the deaths documented during the 1918 influenza pandemic in young individuals were related to a secondary bacterial superinfection, which was commonly by *S. aureus*. In recent years, *S. aureus* isolates that produce the PVL toxin have been associated with skin and soft tissue infection as well as pneumonia in healthy young individuals (15). PVL is rapidly cytolytic to white cells. These strains may also contain other toxins and virulence factors. For these reasons, this infection is associated with a high mortality rate.

Staphylococcus aureus has become over the years, in surprising and unpredictable ways, adapted to new environments and has been able to marshal resistance to almost all of our available antimicrobial agents. Although vancomycin resistance remains an uncommon issue, MRSA poses a serious treatment challenge at the present time. It seems almost a certainty that, at some point, vancomycin-resistant staphylococci will become the next major treatment challenge mounted by this virulent and adaptable organism.

REFERENCES

1. McDonald LC. Trends in antimicrobial resistance in health care-associated pathogens and effect on treatment. Clin Infect Dis 2006; 42(suppl 2):S65–S71.
2. Shorr AF, Tabak YP, Killian AD, Gupta V, Liu LZ, Kollef MH. Healthcare-associated bloodstream infection: a distinct entity? Insights from a large U.S. database. Crit Care Med 2006; 34(10):2588–2595.
3. Kluytmans-Vandenbergh MF, Kluytmans JA. Community-acquired methicillin-resistant *Staphylococcus aureus*: current perspectives. Clin Microbiol Infect 2006; 12(suppl 1):9–15.
4. Diep BA, Sensabaugh GF, Somboona NS, Carleton HA, Perdreau-Remington F. Widespread skin and soft-tissue infections due to two methicillin-resistant *Staphylococcus aureus* strains harboring the genes for Panton–Valentine leucocidin. J Clin Microbiol 2004; 42:2080–2084.
5. National Nosocomial Infections Surveillance (NNIS) System. A report from the National Nosocomial Infections Surveillance System—data summary

from October 1986–April 1996, issued May 1996. Am J Infect Control 1996; 24:380–388.

6. Barrett FF, McGehee RF Jr, Finland M. Methicillin-resistant *Staphylococcus aureus* at Boston City Hospital. Bacteriologic and epidemiologic observations. N Engl J Med 1968; 279:441–448.

7. Crossley K, Landesman B, Zaske D. An outbreak of infections caused by strains of *Staphylococcus aureus* resistant to methicillin and aminoglycosides. II. Epidemiologic studies. J Infect Dis 1979; 139:280–287.

8. Lowy FD. *Staphylococcus aureus* infections. N Engl J Med 1998; 339: 520–532.

9. Noskin GA, Rubin RJ, Schentag JJ, et al. The burden of *Staphylococcus aureus* infections on hospitals in the United States: an analysis of the 2000 and 2001 Nationwide Inpatient Sample Database. Arch Intern Med 2005; 165:1756–1761.

10. Wertheim HF, Melles DC, Vos MC, et al. The role of nasal carriage in *Staphylococcus aureus* infections. Lancet Infect Dis 2005; 5:751–762.

11. Herwaldt LA. *Staphylococcus aureus* nasal carriage and surgical-site infections. Surgery 2003; 134:S2–S9.

12. von Eiff C, Becker K, Machka K, Stammer H, Peters G. Nasal carriage as a source of *Staphylococcus aureus* bacteremia. Study Group. N Engl J Med 2001; 344:11–16.

13. Fowler VG Jr, Miro JM, Hoen B, et al. *Staphylococcus aureus* endocarditis: a consequence of medical progress. JAMA 2005; 293:3012–3021.

14. Habib G, Derumeaux G, Avierinos JF, et al. Value and limitations of the Duke criteria for the diagnosis of infective endocarditis. J Am Coll Cardiol 1999; 33:2023–2029.

15. Francis JS, Doherty MC, Lopatin U, et al. Severe community-onset pneumonia in healthy adults caused by methicillin-resistant *Staphylococcus aureus* carrying the Panton–Valentine leukocidin genes. Clin Infect Dis 2005; 40:100–107.

Epidemiology of MRSA

2

Nasia Safdar and Barry C. Fox
Department of Medicine, University of Wisconsin Medical School
and University of Wisconsin Hospital and Clinics, and the
William S. Middleton Veterans Affairs Medical Center,
Madison, Wisconsin, U.S.A.

Linda M. McKinley
Department of Infection Control, the William S. Middleton
Veterans Affairs Medical Center, Madison, Wisconsin, U.S.A.

INTRODUCTION

Methicillin-resistant *Staphylococcus aureus* (MRSA) is a major cause of infections in healthcare institutions (1) and more recently in the community (2,3). MRSA was first reported in 1961, two years after the introduction of methicillin for treatment of penicillin-resistant *S. aureus* infections (4,5). Despite extensive infection control efforts, methicillin resistance among isolates of *S. aureus* has steadily increased. Data from the National Healthcare-associated Infections Surveillance (NHIS) system of the Centers for Disease Control and Prevention (CDC) show that 50% of healthcare-associated *S. aureus* isolates are now resistant to methicillin. Figure 1 shows resistance trends in *S. aureus* over time (6). Multidrug-resistant strains of staphylococci are also being reported with increasing frequency worldwide, including isolates that are resistant to methicillin, lincosamides, macrolides, aminoglycosides, fluoroquinolones, or combinations of these antibiotics (7). The recent emergence of *S. aureus* strains with intermediate resistance to vancomycin has been reported (8–10). MRSA infections are associated with prolonged hospitalization and increased costs (11,12); some (13,14) but not all (15) studies have

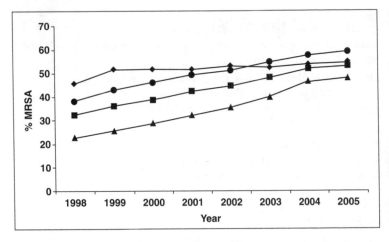

FIGURE 1 MRSA trends (1998–YTD 2005) according to patient location. Data are cumulative for 1998–March 2005. *Key*: ──■──, All patients; ──◆──, ICU patients; ──●──, inpatients; ──▲──, outpatients. *Source*: Adapted from Ref. 6.

also reported excess mortality with MRSA infections. Control of the spread of MRSA in the healthcare setting and in the community is clearly essential. Understanding the natural history and epidemiology of MRSA colonization and infection is fundamental to devising effective strategies for prevention and control.

COLONIZATION WITH *STAPHYLOCOCCUS AUREUS* AND MRSA

Approximately 30% of the population may carry *S. aureus*, usually methicillin-susceptible strains in the nares or on the skin (16). Colonization of the anterior nares with *S. aureus* has been shown to be a risk factor for invasive infection. A recent study found that in 12 of 14 patients the strain causing bacteremia was identical to the strain that had previously been recovered from the anterior nares (17). Determinants of *S. aureus* carriage include host, microbial, and environmental factors.

Studies conducted in acute-care settings show a prevalence of MRSA carriage on admission ranging between 1% and 12% (18–20). As with susceptible strains of *S. aureus*, asymptomatic colonization with MRSA generally precedes infection. In most cases, healthcare-associated infection is a three-step process: (*i*) colonization of the patient's mucosa or skin by a potential pathogen; (*ii*) access of the pathogen to a site where it can invade and produce local infection; and (*iii*) impairment of local host defenses by invasive devices or surgery, fostering invasive infection (21).

Identification of patients likely to be colonized with MRSA on admission is key to promptly deploying contact precautions. Jernigan et al. (22) estimated that the rate of healthcare-associated MRSA (HA-MRSA) transmission was 0.14 transmissions per day; contact precautions lowered this rate sixteen-fold. A number of risk factors for acquisition or carriage of MRSA on admission to an acute care hospital have been enumerated. These are broadly categorized into risk factors intrinsic to the patient, such as gender, older age, and comorbidities, and extrinsic risk factors, such as antimicrobial exposure, use of invasive devices, and the underlying prevalence of MRSA in an institution (23). A protective factor against MRSA colonization is methicillin-sensitive *Staphylococcus aureus* (MSSA) colonization. Dall (24) found that colonization by MSSA protected against colonization by MRSA.

While the dynamics of MRSA carriage are not entirely understood, it is clear that the risk of invasive infection following colonization with MRSA is greater than the risk of infection following colonization with methicillin-susceptible *S. aureus.* MRSA colonization confers a three- to 16-fold increased risk for invasive infection compared with MSSA colonization (18,25–27). The results of these studies are summarized in Table 1.

In the community setting, the prevalence of colonization with MRSA is much lower but is thought to be increasing. A recent study

TABLE 1 Risk of Infection Following Colonization with MRSA Compared with MSSA

No. of patients colonized with MRSA	No. of patients colonized with MSSA	No. of patients infected with MRSA	No. of patients infected with MSSA	OR (95% CI)	Reference
63	84	24	8	5.85 (2.25–16.31)	(26)
26	137	5	2	16.07 (2.37–173.81)	(18)
32	44	8	2	7.0 (1.23–71.06)	(27)
20	141	3	6	3.97 (0.58–20.50)	(25)

Abbreviations: CI, confidence interval; MRSA, methicillin-resistant *Staphylococcus aureus*; MSSA, methicillin-sensitive *Staphylococcus aureus*; OR, odds ratio.

using data from the National Health and Nutrition Examination Survey (NHANES), found that the prevalence of colonization with MRSA was 0.84% in the noninstitutionalized U.S. population (28).

Risk Factors for MRSA Carriage at Admission

Variables reflecting prior contact with the healthcare setting are associated with MRSA carriage on admission. A risk index for predicting patients with MRSA carriage on admission found that the presence of any of the following: age >80 years, previous hospitalization within past 12 months, previous antibiotic use within past six months, and urinary catheter present on admission, would successfully identify the majority of patients with MRSA carriage at admission (29). In a prospective study of 697 patients, Furuno et al. (19) found that patient self-report of a hospital admission in the previous year had a sensitivity of 76% in identifying patients colonized with MRSA. Guidelines from the Healthcare Society for Epidemiology of America recommend screening patients at high risk for MRSA carriage with nasal cultures on admission and periodically throughout hospital stay (30). Contact precautions including the use of a sterile gown and gloves prior to entering the patient's room are instituted for patients found to be colonized. The associated costs are substantial and most healthcare institutions do not routinely screen new admissions for MRSA. The ability to accurately predict a high likelihood of colonization with MRSA at admission would allow the selective application of screening cultures, which could reduce screening costs.

Risk Factors for Acquisition of Healthcare-Associated MRSA

The main modifiable factors that predispose hospitalized patients to acquire colonization or develop infection with MRSA are use of invasive devices, colonization pressure, and antimicrobial exposure.

Use of Indwelling Devices

Invasive devices of all types play a far more important role in increasing susceptibility to healthcare-associated infection than underlying diseases.

Risk factor analysis shows that most healthcare-associated infections, whether caused by resistant or susceptible microorganisms, derive from invasive procedures or invasive devices. The vast majority of HA- MRSA bacteremias are intravascular device-related. More consistent compliance with evidence-based guidelines for prevention of intravascular device-related bloodstream infection (31–33), ventilator-associated pneumonia (34), surgical site infection (35), and catheter-associated urinary tract infection (36,37), as well as novel technology designed for prevention of device-associated infection (32,37) represent potential strategies for containing MRSA in healthcare institutions. However, a wealth of literature shows that translation of evidence into practice is difficult to achieve.

A recent initiative to implement evidence-based guidelines to reduce healthcare-associated device-related infections is found in the Institute for Healthcare Improvement (IHI) 100,000 Lives campaign. This campaign is a national initiative with a goal of saving 100,000 lives among patients in hospitals through improvements in healthcare (38). The initiative assembles interventions into patient care protocols or bundles for which efficacy is documented in the peer-reviewed literature. These bundles group best practices with respect to a disease process that individually improve care and could be additive in their effects when combined. The central line bundle has five key components: (*i*) hand hygiene; (*ii*) maximal barrier precautions; (*iii*) chlorhexidine skin antisepsis; (*iv*) optimal catheter site selection, with subclavian vein as the preferred site for nontunneled catheters; and (*v*) daily review of line necessity, with prompt removal of unnecessary lines. The ventilator bundle has four key components: (*i*) elevation of the head of the bed to between 30° and 45°; (*ii*) daily "sedative interruption" and daily assessment of readiness to extubate; (*iii*) peptic ulcer disease (PUD) prophylaxis; and (*iv*) deep venous thrombosis (DVT) prophylaxis (unless contraindicated). The approach has been most successful when all elements are executed together, an "all or none" strategy.

Colonization Pressure

The prevalence of MRSA colonization or infection in a unit is a powerful risk factor for individual MRSA acquisition in that unit. In a prospective study, Merrer et al. (39) found that weekly colonization pressure (defined as the number of MRSA imported + HA-MRSA patient-days/ total number of patient-days in the week) of 30% or more was associated with a five-fold higher risk of MRSA acquisition. The major mechanism of healthcare-associated transmission of MRSA is from the hands of healthcare workers. Hand hygiene is fundamental to infection control and hand hygiene using waterless alcohol-based handrubs has been shown to reduce nosocomial infections, including those caused by MRSA (40). However, consistent long-term compliance with hand hygiene has been difficult to achieve and many institutions report rates of hand hygiene compliance less than 50%.

Antimicrobial Exposure

Studies highlight the importance of antimicrobial exposure as a risk factor for the acquisition and transmission of MRSA (41). A number of different classes of antimicrobials have been implicated and both overall institutional use and individual patient use of antimicrobials increases the risk of MRSA. Muller et al. (42) attempted to define the relative contribution of institutional antimicrobial use and individual antimicrobial use and found that penicillin use at the hospital level and fluoroquinolone use at the individual level increased the risk of MRSA isolation from a clinical specimen. Other studies confirm an increased risk with fluoroquinolone use (43,44). It is likely that the fluoroquinolone effect is mediated by eradication of MSSA and increased expression of adherence factors, both of which may promote colonization by MRSA (45,46). Whether there are differences among the fluoroquinolones as regards the risk of MRSA colonization or infection is as yet unclear. Table 2 summarizes major studies that have found fluoroquinolone use to be a risk factor for MRSA colonization or infection.

TABLE 2 Fluoroquinolone Exposure as a Risk Factor for MRSA Colonization or Infection

Antimicrobial	Group or individual effect	Estimate of risk	Reference
Penicillins	Group	2.52 (1.15–5.51)	(42)
Fluoroquinolones	Individual	2.63 (1.44–4.80)	
Fluoroquinolones	Group	Statistically significant increase in MRSA colonization or infection with ciprofloxacin and levofloxacin	(44)
Levofloxacin	Individual	3.38 (1.94–5.90)	(43)
Ciprofloxacin	Individual	2.48 (1.32–4.67)	
Levofloxacin	Individual	8.01 (3.15–20.3)	(78)

Abbreviation: MRSA, methicillin-resistant *Staphylococcus aureus*.

Other antimicrobials such as cephalosporins may influence the incidence of MRSA. However, most studies have not made a distinction between the effect of an antibiotic at the group level and that at the individual level. Further research is needed to accurately determine the magnitude of risk associated with various antimicrobials for MRSA.

Co-colonization with Other Multi-Resistant Pathogens

Risk factors for acquisition of carriage or infection by different types of multi-resistant pathogens may be similar (23). In a study of 878 intensive care unit (ICU) patients, 83 (9.5%) were colonized with both MRSA and vancomycin-resistant enterococci (VRE). Co-colonization by VRE and MRSA may facilitate transfer of genes conferring glycopeptide resistance from VRE to MRSA. The recent emergence of vancomycin-resistant *S. aureus* highlights the need for aggressive infection control measures in the institution.

MECHANISMS OF HEALTHCARE-ASSOCIATED TRANSMISSION

Clinical infections by multi-resistant organisms such as MRSA represent the tip of the iceberg of the vast population of colonized patients, most of whom are unrecognized. Colonized patients are the main reservoir of MRSA. For every patient known to be colonized or infected by multi-resistant organisms, a far larger number with unrecognized colonization is already in the institution and, probably, in that patient care unit (47–52).

The major mechanism of patient-to-patient spread of resistant microorganisms is on the hands, equipment or apparel of healthcare workers (53–59). A prospective study found that after performing morning care activities for patients with MRSA in urine or a wound, 65% of nurses cultured showed concordant contamination of their gown or uniform (60).

An epidemiologic study of the spread of MRSA in a university hospital identified roommate-to-roommate transmission and bed-to-adjacent bedspread within an ICU, showing that geographic proximity to an infected or colonized patient greatly increased the risk of acquisition of MRSA (56). Another issue with HA-MRSA is the unique challenges each setting (long-term care, ICU, and ambulatory care) has when implementing precautions; i.e., availability of private rooms, roommate selection, common areas (waiting rooms, dining rooms).

Potential Role of the Inanimate Environment

While the role of environmental contamination in contributing to healthcare-associated infection is unclear, a growing number of studies have found that MRSA may be recovered from hospital equipment and apparatus, such as stethoscopes (61), blood pressure cuffs (62), tourniquets (63), and computer terminals (64). The environment has been implicated in outbreaks of MRSA, which were controlled only after environmental cleaning (65,66). Hardy et al. (67) performed serial environmental and patient screening cultures using selective media and found that MRSA could be recovered from the environment at every sampling; however, only 3 of 26 patients who acquired MRSA in the hospital acquired it from the environment. Sexton et al. (68) reported that the strains of MRSA causing infection in patients were similar to those recovered from the environment in 14 of 20 (70%) patients. The CDC guidelines on hand hygiene recommend hand washing before, in addition to after, patient contact to account for the role of environment in contact transmission (69). No special cleaning protocols are recommended other than the consistent use of a hospital-approved disinfectant.

Community-Acquired MRSA

Until recently, MRSA was, with rare exception, a healthcare-associated pathogen. However, in the last few years, multiple studies have documented cases of MRSA skin and soft tissue infections in persons in the community without traditional risk factors to suggest HA-MRSA. Termed community-associated or community-acquired MRSA (CA-MRSA), these infections are increasing in incidence, and numerous outbreaks in participants of competitive sports (70), children (71), incarcerated persons (72), military recruits (73), and tattoo recipients (74) have been described. Other population groups with high rates of CA-MRSA infections include Alaska natives, Native Americans, and Pacific Islanders.

A report from the CDC Active Bacterial Core Surveillance Program using data from Atlanta, Minnesota, and Baltimore to determine the incidence of endemic CA-MRSA showed that from 2001 through 2002, 1647 cases of CA-MRSA infection were reported, representing between 8% and 20% of all MRSA isolates. The annual disease incidence varied according to site (25.7 cases per 100,000 population in Atlanta vs. 18.0 per 100,000 in Baltimore) and was significantly higher among persons less than two years old than among those who were two years of age or older (relative risk, 1.51; 95% confidence interval, 1.19–1.92) and among blacks than among whites in Atlanta (age-adjusted relative risk, 2.74; 95% confidence interval, 2.44–3.07) (75).

Differences Between Healthcare-Associated and Community-Acquired MRSA

CA-MRSA differs in several ways from HA-MRSA. CA-MRSA is not associated with known risk factors—comorbidities and long-term antibiotic use—and is much more likely than healthcare-associated strains to cause skin and soft tissues infections. CA-MRSA strains carry genes for Panton–Valentine leukocidin, which produce cytotoxins that cause tissue necrosis and leukocyte destruction. While HA-MRSA strains are typically multi-drug-resistant, CA-MRSA strains are susceptible to more classes of drugs (Table 3). PFGE typing shows that the US300 strain of *S. aureus* is responsible for much of the CA-MRSA disease burden in the United States (Fig. 2). Outbreaks of CA-MRSA invasive infection in

TABLE 3 Comparison of Antibiotic Susceptibilities of Healthcare-Associated and Community-Associated MRSA Strains

	No. (%) susceptible		
Antibiotic	Community-associated ($n = 106$)	Healthcare-associated ($n = 211$)	*P*-value
Oxacillin	0	0	NA
Ciprofloxacin	84 (79)	33 (16)	<0.001
Clindamycin	88 (83)	44 (21)	<0.001
Erythromycin	47 (44)	18 (9)	<0.001
Gentamicin	100 (94)	168 (80)	0.001
Rifampin	102 (96)	199 (94)	0.64
Tetracycline	98 (92)	194 (92)	0.95
Trimethoprim-sulfamethoxazole	101 (95)	189 (90)	0.13
Vancomycin	106 (100)	211 (100)	NA

Source: Adapted from Ref. 79.

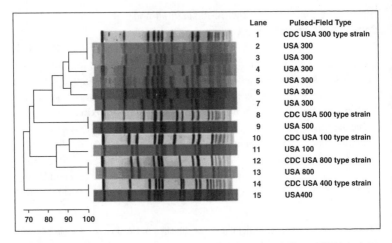

Lane	Pulsed-Field Type
1	CDC USA 300 type strain
2	USA 300
3	USA 300
4	USA 300
5	USA 300
6	USA 300
7	USA 300
8	CDC USA 500 type strain
9	USA 500
10	CDC USA 100 type strain
11	USA 100
12	CDC USA 800 type strain
13	USA 800
14	CDC USA 400 type strain
15	USA400

70   80   90   100

FIGURE 2 Dendrogram of representative pulsed-field types from MRSA isolates causing skin and soft tissue infections. The figure shows infections among patients seen at Grady Memorial Hospital (lanes 2 to 7, 9, 11, 13, and 15) and representative MRSA standard-type strains previously published by the Centers for Disease Control and Prevention (lanes 1, 8, 10, 12, and 14). *Source*: Adapted from Ref. 77.

families are reported (76). Characteristics that are often used to distinguish HA-MRSA and CA-MRSA are summarized in Table 4.

Prevention of CA-MRSA transmission in the community uses similar tactics as those used in the hospital setting: hand hygiene and proper wound care at simple effective interventions. More specific recommendations are not available.

CONCLUSION

In conclusion, MRSA is a major cause of healthcare-associated infections and is emerging as the major cause of skin and soft tissue infections in the community. Colonization of the anterior nares usually precedes infection.

TABLE 4 Risk Factors for Community-Acquired MRSA

Factor	HA-MRSA	CA-MRSA
Risk factors and at-risk populations	Previous contact with healthcare settings	Team-sport participants, incarcerated persons, military, and children
SCC type	Type II	Type IV
PFGE type	US 100	US 300
Toxins	Fewer	More
PVL	Rare	Common
Antibiotic resistance pattern	Multiply resistant	Sensitive to many except beta-lactams
Associated clinical syndromes	Bacteremia, pneumonia	Skin and soft tissue infections

Abbreviations: CA-MRSA, community-acquired methicillin-resistant *Staphylococcus aureus*; HA-MRSA, healthcare-associated methicillin-resistant *Staphylococcus aureus*; PFGE, pulsed field gel electrophoresis; PVL, Panton–Valentine leukocidin; SCC, staphylococcal cassette chromosome.

Colonized patients represent the major institutional reservoir of MRSA. Healthcare-associated transmission of MRSA occurs from the hands, equipment, and apparel of healthcare workers.

Colonization pressure and antimicrobial exposure are important risk factors for healthcare-associated acquisition of MRSA. Groups at high risk for CA-MRSA include children, persons incarcerated or in the military, and participants in team sports. Knowledge of the epidemiology of MRSA will enhance our ability to develop measures to contain it.

REFERENCES

1. Panlilio AL, Culver DH, Gaynes RP, et al. Methicillin-resistant *Staphylococcus aureus* in U.S. hospitals, 1975–1991. Infect Control Hosp Epidemiol 1992; 13:582–586.

2. Drews TD, Temte JL, Fox BC. Community-associated methicillin-resistant *Staphylococcus aureus*: review of an emerging public health concern. WMJ 2006; 105:52–57.

3. Vandenesch F, Naimi T, Enright MC, et al. Community-acquired methicillin-resistant *Staphylococcus aureus* carrying Panton-Valentine leukocidin genes: worldwide emergence. Emerg Infect Dis 2003; 9:978–984.

4. Enright MC, Robinson DA, Randle G, et al. The evolutionary history of methicillin-resistant *Staphylococcus aureus* (MRSA). Proc Natl Acad Sci USA 2002; 99:7687–7692.

5. Jevons MP, Coe AW, Parker MT. Methicillin resistance in staphylococci. Lancet 1963; 1:904–907.

6. Styers D, Sheehan DJ, Hogan P, et al. Laboratory-based surveillance of current antimicrobial resistance patterns and trends among *Staphylococcus aureus*: 2005 status in the United States. Ann Clin Microbiol Antimicrob 2006; 5:2.

7. Deshpande LM, Fritsche TR, Jones RN. Molecular epidemiology of selected multidrug-resistant bacteria: a global report from the sentry antimicrobial surveillance program. Diagn Microbiol Infect Dis 2004; 49:231–236.

8. Chang S, Sievert DM, Hageman JC, et al. Infection with vancomycin-resistant *Staphylococcus aureus* containing the vanA resistance gene. N Engl J Med 2003; 348:1342–1347.

9. Sieradzki K, Roberts RB, Haber SW, et al. The development of vancomycin resistance in a patient with methicillin-resistant *Staphylococcus aureus* infection. N Engl J Med 1999; 340:517–523.

10. Smith TL, Pearson ML, Wilcox KR, et al. Emergence of vancomycin resistance in *Staphylococcus aureus*. Glycopeptide-intermediate *Staphylococcus aureus* working group. N Engl J Med 1999; 340:493–501.

11. Cosgrove SE, Qi Y, Kaye KS, et al. The impact of methicillin resistance in *Staphylococcus aureus* bacteremia on patient outcomes: mortality, length of stay, and hospital charges. Infect Control Hosp Epidemiol 2005; 26:166–174.

12. Engemann JJ, Carmeli Y, Cosgrove SE, et al. Adverse clinical and economic outcomes attributable to methicillin resistance among patients with *Staphylococcus aureus* surgical site infection. Clin Infect Dis 2003; 36: 592–598.

13. Chang FY, MacDonald BB, Peacock JE Jr, et al. A prospective multicenter study of *Staphylococcus aureus* bacteremia: incidence of endocarditis, risk factors for mortality, and clinical impact of methicillin resistance. Medicine (Baltimore) 2003; 82:322–332.

14. Ridenour GA, Wong ES, Call MA, et al. Duration of colonization with methicillin-resistant *Staphylococcus aureus* among patients in the intensive care unit: implications for intervention. Infect Control Hosp Epidemiol 2006; 27:271–278.
15. Zahar JR, Clec'h C, Tafflet M, et al. Is methicillin resistance associated with a worse prognosis in *Staphylococcus aureus* ventilator-associated pneumonia? Clin Infect Dis 2005; 41:1224–1231.
16. Wertheim HF, Melles DC, Vos MC, et al. The role of nasal carriage in *Staphylococcus aureus* infections. Lancet Infect Dis 2005; 5:751–762.
17. von Eiff C, Becker K, Machka K, et al. Nasal carriage as a source of *Staphylococcus aureus* bacteremia. Study Group. N Engl J Med 2001; 344:11–16.
18. Davis KA, Stewart JJ, Crouch HK, et al. Methicillin-resistant *Staphylococcus aureus* (MRSA) nares colonization at hospital admission and its effect on subsequent MRSA infection. Clin Infect Dis 2004; 39:776–782.
19. Furuno JP, Harris AD, Wright MO, et al. Prediction rules to identify patients with methicillin-resistant *Staphylococcus aureus* and vancomycin-resistant enterococci upon hospital admission. Am J Infect Control 2004; 32:436–440.
20. Samad A, Banerjee D, Carbarns N, et al. Prevalence of methicillin-resistant *Staphylococcus aureus* colonization in surgical patients, on admission to a Welsh hospital. J Hosp Infect 2002; 51:43–46.
21. Bonten MJ, Weinstein RA. The role of colonization in the pathogenesis of nosocomial infections. Infect Control Hosp Epidemiol 1996; 17:193–200.
22. Jernigan JA, Titus MG, Groschel DH, et al. Effectiveness of contact isolation during a hospital outbreak of methicillin-resistant *Staphylococcus aureus*. Am J Epidemiol 1996; 143:496–504.
23. Safdar N, Maki DG. The commonality of risk factors for nosocomial colonization and infection with antimicrobial-resistant *Staphylococcus aureus*, enterococcus, gram-negative bacilli, *Clostridium difficile*, and Candida. Ann Intern Med 2002; 136:834–844.
24. Dall'Antonia M, Coen PG, Wilks M, et al. Competition between methicillin-sensitive and -resistant *Staphylococcus aureus* in the anterior nares. J Hosp Infect 2005; 61:62–67.
25. Fishbain JT, Lee JC, Nguyen HD, et al. Nosocomial transmission of methicillin-resistant *Staphylococcus aureus*: a blinded study to establish baseline acquisition rates. Infect Control Hosp Epidemiol 2003; 24:415–421.
26. Pujol M, Pena C, Pallares R, et al. Nosocomial *Staphylococcus aureus* bacteremia among nasal carriers of methicillin-resistant and methicillin-susceptible strains. Am J Med 1996; 100:509–516.

27. Muder RR, Brennen C, Wagener MM, et al. Methicillin-resistant staphylococcal colonization and infection in a long-term care facility. Ann Intern Med 1991; 114:107–112.

28. Graham PL III, Lin SX, Larson EL. A U.S. population-based survey of *Staphylococcus aureus* colonization. Ann Intern Med 2006; 144:318–325.

29. Harbarth S, Sax H, Fankhauser-Rodriguez C, et al. Evaluating the probability of previously unknown carriage of MRSA at hospital admission. Am J Med 2006; 119:275 e15–e23.

30. Muto CA, Jernigan JA, Ostrowsky BE, et al. SHEA guideline for preventing nosocomial transmission of multidrug-resistant strains of *Staphylococcus aureus* and enterococcus. Infect Control Hosp Epidemiol 2003; 24:362–386.

31. O'Grady NP, Alexander M, Dellinger EP, et al. Guidelines for the prevention of intravascular catheter-related infections. Centers for Disease Control and Prevention. MMWR Recomm Rep 2002; 51:1–29.

32. Crnich CJ, Maki DG. The promise of novel technology for the prevention of intravascular device-related bloodstream infection. I. Pathogenesis and short-term devices. Clin Infect Dis 2002; 34:1232–1242.

33. Crnich CJ, Maki DG. The promise of novel technology for the prevention of intravascular device-related bloodstream infection. II. Long-term devices. Clin Infect Dis 2002; 34:1362–1368.

34. Tablan OC, Anderson LJ, Besser R, et al. Guidelines for preventing health-care-associated pneumonia, 2003: recommendations of CDC and the health-care infection control practices advisory committee. MMWR Recomm Rep 2004; 53:1–36.

35. Mangram AJ, Horan TC, Pearson ML, et al. Guideline for prevention of surgical site infection, 1999. Centers for Disease Control and Prevention (CDC) hospital infection control practices advisory committee. Am J Infect Control 1999; 27:97–132; quiz 133–134; discussion 96.

36. Wong ES. Guideline for prevention of catheter-associated urinary tract infections. Am J Infect Control 1983; 11:28–36.

37. Maki DG, Tambyah PA. Engineering out the risk for infection with urinary catheters. Emerg Infect Dis 2001; 7:342–347.

38. Berwick DM, Calkins DR, McCannon CJ, et al. The 100,000 lives campaign: setting a goal and a deadline for improving health care quality. J Am Med Assoc 2006; 295:324–327.

39. Merrer J, Santoli F, Appere de Vecchi C, et al. "Colonization pressure" and risk of acquisition of methicillin-resistant *Staphylococcus aureus* in a medical intensive care unit. Infect Control Hosp Epidemiol 2000; 21:718–723.

40. Pittet D, Hugonnet S, Harbarth S, et al. Effectiveness of a hospital-wide programme to improve compliance with hand hygiene. Infection Control Programme. Lancet 2000; 356:1307–1312.

41. Muller AA, Mauny F, Bertin M, et al. Relationship between spread of methicillin-resistant *Staphylococcus aureus* and antimicrobial use in a French university hospital. Clin Infect Dis 2003; 36:971–978.

42. Muller A, Mauny F, Talon D, et al. Effect of individual- and group-level antibiotic exposure on MRSA isolation: a multilevel analysis. J Antimicrob Chemother 2006 (submitted for publication).

43. Weber SG, Gold HS, Hooper DC, et al. Fluoroquinolones and the risk for methicillin-resistant *Staphylococcus aureus* in hospitalized patients. Emerg Infect Dis 2003; 9:1415–1422.

44. Bosso JA, Mauldin PD. Using interrupted time series analysis to assess associations of fluoroquinolone formulary changes with susceptibility of gram-negative pathogens and isolation rates of methicillin-resistant *Staphylococcus aureus*. Antimicrob Agents Chemother 2006; 50:2106–2112.

45. Bisognano C, Vaudaux P, Rohner P, et al. Induction of fibronectin-binding proteins and increased adhesion of quinolone-resistant *Staphylococcus aureus* by subinhibitory levels of ciprofloxacin. Antimicrob Agents Chemother 2000; 44:1428–1437.

46. Bisognano C, Vaudaux PE, Lew DP, et al. Increased expression of fibronectin-binding proteins by fluoroquinolone-resistant *Staphylococcus aureus* exposed to subinhibitory levels of ciprofloxacin. Antimicrob Agents Chemother 1997; 41:906–913.

47. Martone WJ. Spread of vancomycin-resistant enterococci: why did it happen in the United States? Infect Control Hosp Epidemiol 1998; 19:539–545.

48. Tucci V, Haran MA, Isenberg HD. Epidemiology and control of vancomycin-resistant enterococci in an adult and children's hospital. Am J Infect Control 1997; 25:371–376.

49. Pegues DA, Pegues CF, Hibberd PL, et al. Emergence and dissemination of a highly vancomycin-resistant vanA strain of *Enterococcus faecium* at a large teaching hospital. J Clin Microbiol 1997; 35:1565–1570.

50. Boyce JM, Opal SM, Chow JW, et al. Outbreak of multidrug-resistant *Enterococcus faecium* with transferable vanB class vancomycin resistance. J Clin Microbiol 1994; 32:1148–1153.

51. Montecalvo MA, Jarvis WR, Uman J, et al. Infection-control measures reduce transmission of vancomycin-resistant enterococci in an endemic setting. Ann Intern Med 1999; 131:269–272.

52. Quale J, Landman D, Atwood E, et al. Experience with a hospital-wide outbreak of vancomycin-resistant enterococci. Am J Infect Control 1996; 24: 372–379.

53. Knittle MA, Eitzman DV, Baer H. Role of hand contamination of personnel in the epidemiology of gram-negative nosocomial infections. J Pediatr 1975; 86:433–437.

54. Handwerger S, Raucher B, Altarac D, et al. Nosocomial outbreak due to *Enterococcus faecium* highly resistant to vancomycin, penicillin, and gentamicin. Clin Infect Dis 1993; 16:750–755.

55. Zachary KC, Bayne PS, Morrison VJ, et al. Contamination of gowns, gloves, and stethoscopes with vancomycin-resistant enterococci. Infect Control Hosp Epidemiol 2001; 22:560–564.

56. Peacock JE Jr, Marsik FJ, Wenzel RP. Methicillin-resistant *Staphylococcus aureus*: introduction and spread within a hospital. Ann Intern Med 1980; 93:526–532.

57. Thompson RL, Cabezudo I, Wenzel RP. Epidemiology of nosocomial infections caused by methicillin-resistant *Staphylococcus aureus*. Ann Intern Med 1982; 97:309–317.

58. Crossley K, Landesman B, Zaske D. An outbreak of infections caused by strains of *Staphylococcus aureus* resistant to methicillin and aminoglycosides. II. Epidemiologic studies. J Infect Dis 1979; 139:280–287.

59. Crossley K, Loesch D, Landesman B, et al. An outbreak of infections caused by strains of *Staphylococcus aureus* resistant to methicillin and aminoglycosides. I. Clinical studies. J Infect Dis 1979; 139:273–279.

60. Boyce JM, Chenevert C. Isolation gowns prevent health care workers (HCWs) from contaminating their clothing, and possibly their hands, with methicillin-resistant *Staphylococcus aureus* (MRSA) and resistant enterococci. The Eighth Annual Meeting of the Society for Healthcare Epidemiology of America. Orlando, FL: 1998:72.

61. Cohen HA, Amir J, Matalon A, et al. Stethoscopes and otoscopes—a potential vector of infection? Fam Pract 1997; 14:446–449.

62. Layton MC, Perez M, Heald P, et al. An outbreak of mupirocin-resistant *Staphylococcus aureus* on a dermatology ward associated with an environmental reservoir. Infect Control Hosp Epidemiol 1993; 14:369–375.

63. Berman DS, Schaefler S, Simberkoff MS, et al. Tourniquets and nosocomial methicillin-resistant *Staphylococcus aureus* infections. N Engl J Med 1986; 315:514–515.

64. Devine J, Cooke RP, Wright EP. Is methicillin-resistant *Staphylococcus aureus* (MRSA) contamination of ward-based computer terminals a surrogate marker

for nosocomial MRSA transmission and hand washing compliance? J Hosp Infect 2001; 48:72–75.

65. Embil JM, McLeod JA, Al-Barrak AM, et al. An outbreak of methicillin resistant *Staphylococcus aureus* on a burn unit: potential role of contaminated hydrotherapy equipment. Burns 2001; 27:681–688.

66. Kumari DN, Haji TC, Keer V, et al. Ventilation grilles as a potential source of methicillin-resistant *Staphylococcus aureus* causing an outbreak in an orthopaedic ward at a district general hospital. J Hosp Infect 1998; 39:127–133.

67. Hardy KJ, Oppenheim BA, Gossain S, et al. A study of the relationship between environmental contamination with methicillin-resistant *Staphylococcus aureus* (MRSA) and patients' acquisition of MRSA. Infect Control Hosp Epidemiol 2006; 27:127–132.

68. Sexton T, Clarke P, O'Neill E, et al. Environmental reservoirs of methicillin-resistant *Staphylococcus aureus* in isolation rooms: correlation with patient isolates and implications for hospital hygiene. J Hosp Infect 2006; 62:187–194.

69. Boyce JM, Pittet D. Guideline for hand hygiene in health-care settings. Recommendations of the Healthcare Infection Control Practices Advisory Committee and the HICPAC/SHEA/APIC/IDSA Hand Hygiene Task Force. Society for Healthcare Epidemiology of America/Association for Professionals in Infection Control/Infectious Diseases Society of America. MMWR Recomm Rep 2002; 51:1–45; quiz CE1-4.

70. Kazakova SV, Hageman JC, Matava M, et al. A clone of methicillin-resistant *Staphylococcus aureus* among professional football players. N Engl J Med 2005; 352:468–475.

71. Herold BC, Immergluck LC, Maranan MC, et al. Community-acquired methicillin-resistant *Staphylococcus aureus* in children with no identified predisposing risk. J Am Med Assoc 1998; 279:593–598.

72. Methicillin-resistant *Staphylococcus aureus* infections in correctional facilities—Georgia, California, and Texas, 2001–2003. MMWR Morb Mortal Wkly Rep 2003; 52:992–996.

73. Campbell KM, Vaughn AF, Russell KL, et al. Risk factors for community-associated methicillin-resistant *Staphylococcus aureus* infections in an outbreak of disease among military trainees in San Diego, California, in 2002. J Clin Microbiol 2004; 42:4050–4053.

74. Methicillin-resistant *Staphylococcus aureus* skin infections among tattoo recipients—Ohio, Kentucky, and Vermont, 2004–2005. MMWR Morb Mortal Wkly Rep 2006; 55:677–679.

75. Fridkin SK, Hageman JC, Morrison M, et al. Methicillin-resistant *Staphylococcus aureus* disease in three communities. N Engl J Med 2005; 352: 1436–1444.

76. Huijsdens XW, van Santen-Verheuvel MG, Spalburg E, et al. Multiple cases of familial transmission of community-acquired methicillin-resistant *Staphylococcus aureus*. J Clin Microbiol 2006; 44:2994–2996.

77. King MD, Humphrey BJ, Wang YF, et al. Emergence of community-acquired methicillin-resistant *Staphylococcus aureus* USA 300 clone as the predominant cause of skin and soft-tissue infections. Ann Intern Med 2006; 144:309–317.

78. Graffunder EM, Venezia RA. Risk factors associated with nosocomial methicillin-resistant *Staphylococcus aureus* (MRSA) infection including previous use of antimicrobials. J Antimicrob Chemother 2002; 49:999–1005.

79. Naimi TS, LeDell KH, Como-Sabetti K, et al. Comparison of community- and health care-associated methicillin-resistant *Staphylococcus aureus* infection. J Am Med Assoc 2003; 290:2976–2984.

Genetics of MRSA: The United States and Worldwide

Dennis Stevens

Infectious Diseases Section, Veterans Affairs Medical Center,
Boise, Idaho, and Department of Medicine, University of Washington,
Seattle, Washington, U.S.A.

INTRODUCTION

Staphylococcus aureus is once again re-emerging as a major threat to
human health and well-being the world over. With the evolution of man
and medicine, *S. aureus* too has evolved and adapted to a wide variety
of human conditions and medical innovations. Historically, *S. aureus*
was certainly a significant human pathogen prior to the development of
antibiotics. For example, in the last century, *S. aureus* was the major
bacterial cause of death in the influenza pandemic of 1918, among those
who developed secondary bacterial pneumonia. Following the introduction of antibiotics, *S. aureus* developed resistance to penicillin in the
1940s, and then emerged as an important cause of serious nosocomial
infections in the 1950s. With the development and widespread use of
chloramphenicol and tetracycline in the 1960s, superinfections due to
S. aureus occurred, including staphylococcal enterocolitis. These were
clearly related to two factors: antibiotic eradication of the normal gut
flora and concomitant proliferation of *S. aureus* strains, which had
developed antibiotic resistance during treatment. The timely discovery
of beta-lactamase-resistant cephalosporins and later the semisynthetic
beta-lactam antibiotics (methicillin, oxacillin, and nafcillin) saved the

day for the next 10 to 15 years. Still, as early as the 1970s, sporadic reports of methicillin-resistant *S. aureus* (MRSA) began to appear. Epidemics of MRSA were reported in some unique facilities with extremely ill patients and with intense antibiotic usage (1). Over the subsequent 20 to 30 years, we have seen the widespread emergence of MRSA infections in certain regions of Europe, throughout the United States, as well as in Japan and the Western Pacific. Until very recently, these MRSA strains have largely been associated with hospital-acquired infections (HA-MRSA) (2,3).

COMMUNITY-ACQUIRED MRSA: GENETIC DIFFERENCES

Only recently have reports of true community-acquired MRSA (CA-MRSA) infections begun to emerge (4–6). Empiric treatment of some of these with conventional agents was inadequate and resulted in disastrous outcomes before it was determined that the etiologic agent was MRSA (7). There are two lessons to be learned from these dramatic cases. First, these infections did not respond to the types of agents that most of us would prescribe for community-acquired *S. aureus* infections. Second, these were particularly severe types of infection as they resulted in deaths. Thus, these CA-MRSA strains were unique not only because of methicillin-resistance, but also because they were highly virulent. Epidemiologic studies using molecular tools have provided great insight into these infections. These studies are replacing classical epidemiology, which had concluded that these cases must have had some type of contact with healthcare facilities, occult antibiotic exposure, or contact with someone with HA-MRSA. Pulsed gel electrophoresis comparing strains from the community and those from hospital-associated infection demonstrated that multiple different strains were causing the hospital-associated infections, whereas there was an identical pattern for CA-MRSA from diverse infections and from widely disparate geographical areas (8). This pattern has been named the USA100 strain.

Similarly, there is now clear genetic-based evidence that CA-MRSA strains are distinct from HA-MRSA (8,9). In fact, Daum et al. (9) demonstrated that there are at least four different types of *mecA* (methicillin resistance) gene cassettes. Interestingly, types I, II, and III are associated with strains causing HA-MRSA infections, whereas type IV distinguishes CA-MRSA infections. The type IV *mecA* gene cassette is much smaller (23 kD) compared to types I, II, and III that are 95, 80, and 55 kD, respectively. If smaller size is in fact associated with greater likelihood of transfer to sensitive strains, then many strains of *S. aureus* in the community could acquire *mecA* gene cassette type IV and the prevalence of CA-MRSA infections should increase dramatically. Indeed, this phenomenon has come to fruition, and recent estimates document that 59% of staphylococcal species causing skin and soft tissue infections in the outpatient setting are in fact CA-MRSA (10).

Additional reports document an increasing frequency of CA-MRSA infections in the pediatric population (4–7). Based upon the striking similarity patterns of the USA300 strains of CA-MRSA, these have been referred to as a clone. It seems likely that the origin of USA300 was a methicillin-sensitive *S. aureus* (MSSA) strain, probably phage type 80/81, which acquired the type IV *mecA* gene. In fact, with more refined genetic analysis, there are likely many different MSSA strains that have acquired the type IV *mecA* gene (Robert Daum, personal communication). Thus, there are likely multiple unique strains of CA-MRSA throughout the United States.

Unique Syndromes Caused by Toxin-Producing Strains of *Staphylococcus aureus*

Although the adaptability of *S. aureus* to antibiotics is well documented, the acquisition and expression of virulence genes has not been extensively studied. Still, we are well aware historically of the emergence of novel clinical syndromes such as staphylococcal scalded skin syndrome (SSSS), staphylococcal toxic shock syndrome (staph TSS), staphylococcal food poisoning, and more recently necrotizing fasciitis (11) and hemorrhagic necrotizing pneumonia (12). In each case, these novel syndromes have been the result of acquiring mobile genetic elements, usually bacteriophages with subsequent expression of specific extra-cellular toxins.

Staphylococcus aureus: Genetic Elements, Surface Components, and Extracellular Toxins

To understand the complexity of MRSA colonization and infection at the present time, it is important to have a perspective on the genetics, surface structures, metabolism, and extracellular virulence factors of *S. aureus*, which contribute to the bacteria's pathogenesis.

Staphylococci are nonsporulating, nonmotile gram-positive cocci that have an average diameter of 1 μm and microscopically appear as grapelike clusters. When grown on blood agar, staphylococci form small (1 to 2 mm), smooth, round colonies that are often pigmented and may be surrounded by a zone of β-hemolysis. Staphylococci are very hardy organisms and can withstand much more physical and chemical stress than pneumococci and streptococci. For example, staphylococci resist drying, withstand 10% NaCl, and will survive and even replicate at temperatures between 10° and 45°C. Because staphylococci are facultative anaerobes, they will grow in the presence or absence of oxygen.

The cellular structure of *S. aureus* is complex. Most strains have poly-saccharide microcapsules. The cell wall of *S. aureus* is structurally similar to that of Group A streptococci: both have a carbohydrate antigen, a protein component, and a mucopeptide. The carbohydrate antigen is a teichoic acid, which in *S. aureus* is a polymer of *N*-acetylglucosamine and polyri-bitol phosphate. Antibodies to teichoic acid can be detected in normal human serum, and elevated antibody titers are present in patients with deep-seated staphylococcal infections. Teichoic acid has no established role in virulence, and antibodies to this carbohydrate are not protective. The protein component of the cell wall includes protein A, which reacts with IgG of normal human serum (13). Protein A interacts with the Fc component rather than the Fab component of IgG and hence is not a true antigen. Protein A may be antiphagocytic, but its role in virulence has not been clearly established. The cell wall mucopeptide of staphylococci is structurally similar to the mucopeptide of other gram-positive bacteria.

Most strains of *S. aureus* produce a variety of extracellular products, including both enzymes and toxins that may account for the tendency to produce burrowing, destructive, localized infections. The enzyme coagulase causes plasma to clot, thus promoting the fibrin meshwork that contributes to abscess formation. Staphylococci can also produce lipase, protease, hyaluronidase, and DNAse, which can add to tissue damage. Another important enzyme is penicillinase. Because penicillinase has no role in pathogenicity, staphylococci that produce penicillinase are no more virulent than nonpenicillinase-producing strains. Nevertheless, this enzyme is clinically and epidemiologically important, because it hydrolyzes the beta-lactam ring of penicillin, thereby inactivating the molecule. The production of penicillinase is controlled by plasmids, or episomes, which are extrachromosomal DNA molecules that replicate during cell division. Unlike the R factors of gram-negative bacilli, however, the plasmids responsible for penicillinase production do not usually mediate resistance to multiple antibiotics.

Of even greater interest are the nonenzymatic toxins produced by *S. aureus*. α-Toxin is a cytotoxin that produces pores in cell membranes, thereby altering their permeability and resulting in cell damage or death. α-Toxin damages red and white blood cells and activates platelets. Injection of α-toxin into animals can produce dermal necrosis and contraction of vascular smooth muscle, leading to tissue ischemia. Another potential virulence factor is leukocidin, which consists of two leukotoxic proteins that are capable of disrupting lysosomal membranes (14–17). Occasionally, strains of staphylococci produce exfoliatin that causes the epidermolysis of SSSS. Some strains of staphylococci can also produce one of four antigenically distinct enterotoxins that cause the vomiting and diarrhea characteristic of staphylococcal food poisoning. In rare instances, staphylococci produce an erythrogenic toxin that causes scarlet fever. Finally, a staphylococcal exotoxin, toxic-shock syndrome toxin–1 (TSST-1), appears to be responsible for staph TSS.

Pathogenesis of Staphylococcal Infections

The earliest tissue response in staphylococcal infection is acute inflammation with a vigorous exudation of polymorphonuclear leukocytes. Vascular thrombosis and tissue necrosis quickly lead to abscess formation. As a result of the development of a fibrin meshwork and later fibroblast proliferation, these abscesses become walled-off zones of loculated infection and tissue destruction, with dying leukocytes and viable bacteria at the center. Fibrosis and scarring are often prominent in healing.

The importance of the granulocyte in host defense is supported by the enhanced susceptibility to staphylococcal infections seen in patients with neutropenia or various disorders of neutrophil function, such as chronic granulomatous disease, Chédiak-Higashi syndrome, and various disorders of chemotaxis. The most important factors predisposing to staphylococcal infections are not immunologic defects but mechanical defects. Minute skin abrasions, for example, probably provide the portal of entry in staphylococcal skin infections and in many cases of staphylococcal bacteremia. Intravenous drug abuse accounts for many cases of staphylococcal bacteremia and endocarditis. Indwelling venous catheters are particularly important in nosocomial infections; plastic catheters become coated with fibrinogen and fibrin, which interact with adhesions on the bacterial cell surface and bind staphylococci to the catheter.

ARE COMMUNITY-ACQUIRED MRSA STRAINS MORE VIRULENT?

A major concern is the increased potential for more serious CA-MRSA infections. Some investigations have demonstrated a two-fold increase in the prevalence of TSST-1 and staphylococcal enterotoxin in MRSA strains compared to MSSA strains (11). In fact, recent reports from Japan suggest an increase in the frequency of staph TSS caused by MRSA (12–14). In addition, the propensity of MRSA to cause more severe soft tissue infections is suggested by the fatal cases recently reported from the Midwest of the United States (6), by the reports of necrotizing fasciitis caused by CA-MRSA and by fulminant necrotizing hemorrhagic pneumonia following influenza. Similarly, severe staphylococcal infections in France have been reported to be associated with the Panton–Valentine leukocidin (PVL) (17–21). Recent studies in the United States have shown that this toxin is found in 77% of CA-MRSA strains compared to 14% of HA-MRSA and 0% of methicillin-sensitive strains (22), including bacteremia, pneumonia, and soft tissue infections. It has been accepted that MSSA strains rarely produce PVL toxin, yet recent data suggest that one third of MSSA strains produced PVL (23). PVL was almost twice as likely to be found in MRSA strains in this same study, but the 38% prevalence of PVL production by MSSA strains is certainly bothersome. In the future staph TSS may not be limited to menstrual cases or postsurgical cases involving packing material. In addition, pneumonia may be more severe based upon recent studies in France (15–17). Finally, necrotizing soft tissue infections may become more common due to the presence of the PVL (15–17).

SPECIFIC CONSIDERATIONS IN THE SELECTION OF SPECIFIC ANTI-MRSA ANTIMICROBIAL AGENTS

Skin and Soft Tissue Infections

Numerous clinical trials have documented the efficacy of linezolid, vancomycin, daptomycin, quinupristin–dalfopristin, and glycycline in skin and soft tissue infections (22,24).

Pneumonia

There may be some advantage for linezolid due to its excellent penetration into lung alveolar fluid (25). Daptomycin should not be used to treat bacterial pneumonia due to its high protein binding and inactivation by surfactant. Tigecycline has not yet been studied in the treatment of pneumonia.

Bacteremia and Endocarditis

Linezolid and vancomycin have been equivalent in treatment of MRSA-related bacteremia (22), and daptomycin has been shown to be non-inferior to vancomycin for right-sided endocarditis (26). There have been numerous papers describing failures with vancomycin, and agents superior to vancomycin are sorely needed for the treatment of MRSA endocarditis (27).

Toxin-Related Staphylococcal Infections

Necrotizing fasciitis, necrotizing-hemorrhaghic pneumonia, toxic shock syndrome, and scalded skin syndrome: There has never been a clinical trial that specifically addresses antibiotic treatment of staph TSS, thus we are left to base treatment upon in vitro susceptibility data. In addition, suppression of toxin production has been demonstrated with clindamycin and linezolid, and these may offer an advantage in treating patients with toxic shock syndrome. It should be noted that this recommendation is based solely on in vitro toxin suppression data, extrapolation from experimental necrotizing infections caused by Group A streptococcus and *Clostridium perfringens* (Clostridium and GAS models), retrospective analysis, and recently case reports. The true pathogenesis of necrotizing fasciitis and necrotizing pneumonia has not been elucidated, but is associated with CA-MRSA strains producing the PVL. Whether that toxin singly or in combination with other toxins is responsible is being actively studied. Most would agree, however that extracellular toxins play a major role. As such, antibiotics that are capable of suppressing these toxins could provide an added advantage in the treatment of these MRSA infections.

REFERENCES

1. Everett ED, McNitt TR, Rahm AE, Stevens DL, Peterson HE. Epidemiologic investigation of methicillin resistant *Staphylococcus aureus* in a burn unit. Military Med 1978; March:165–167.
2. Graffunder EM, Venezia RA. Risk factors associated with nosocomial methicillin-resistant *Staphylococcus aureus* (MRSA) infection including previous use of antimicrobials. J Antimicrob Chemother 2002; 49:999–1005.
3. Kotilainen P, Routamaa M, Peltonen R, et al. Elimination of epidemic methicillin-resistant *Staphylococcus aureus* from a university hospital and district institutions, Finland. Emerg Infect Dis 2003; 9:169–175.
4. Campbell A, Bryant K, Stover B, Condra C, Marshall GY. Epidemiology of *Staphylococcus aureus* infection at a children's hospital. In: Program & Abstracts of the 40th Annual Infectious Disease Society of America meeting. Chicago, IL, 2002:620.
5. Dietrich DW, Auld DB, Mermel L. Pediatric community-acquired methicillin-resistant *Staphylococcus aureus* in southeastern New England. In: Program & Abstracts of the 40th Annual Infectious Disease Society of America meeting. Chicago, IL, 2002:617.
6. Purcell RK, Fergie JE. Exponential increase in community-acquired MRSA infections in South Texas children. In: Program & Abstracts of the 40th Annual Infectious Disease Society of America meeting. Chicago, IL, 2002:618.
7. Centers for Disease Control: From the Centers for Disease Control and Prevention. Four pediatric deaths from community-acquired methicillin-resistant *Staphylococcus aureus*—Minnesota and North Dakota, 1997–1999. JAMA 1999; 282:1123–1125.
8. Charlebois IE, Perdreau-Remington F. Molecular evidence for clonal distinction between community and nosocomial methicillin-resistant *Staphylococcus aureus* in 536 clinical infections. In: Program & Abstracts of the 40th Annual Infectious Disease Society of America meeting. Chicago, IL, 2002:23.
9. Daum RS, Ito T, Hiramatsu K, et al. A novel methicillin-resistance cassette in community-acquired methicillin-resistant *Staphylococcus aureus* isolates of diverse genetic backgrounds. J Infect Dis 2002; 186:1344–1347.
10. Moran GJ, Krishnadasan A, Gorwitz RJ, et al. Methicillin-resistant *S. aureus* infections among patients in the emergency department. New Engl J Med 2006; 355(7):666–674.

11. Miller LG, Perdreau-Remington F, Rieg G, et al. Necrotizing fasciitis caused by community-associated methicillin-resistant *Staphylococcus aureus* in Los Angeles. N Engl J Med 2005; 352(14):1445–1453.

12. Francis JS, Doherty MC, Lopatin U, et al. Severe community-onset pneumonia in healthy adults caused by methicillin-resistant *Staphylococcus aureus* carrying the Panton-Valentine leukocidin genes. Clin Inf Dis 2005; 40(1):100–107.

13. Lowy FD. *Staphylococcus aureus* infections. N Engl J Med 1998; 339:520.

14. Dufour P, Gillet Y, Bes M, et al. Community-acquired methicillin-resistant *Staphylococcus aureus* infections in France: emergence of a single clone that produces Panton-Valentine leukocidin. Clin Infect Dis 2002; 35:819–824.

15. Gillet Y, Issartel B, Vanhems P, et al. Association between *Staphylococcus aureus* strains carrying gene for Panton-Valentine leukocidin and highly lethal necrotising pneumonia in young immunocompetent patients. Lancet 2002; 359:753–759.

16. Lina F, Piemont Y, Godail-Gamot F, et al. Involvement of Panton-Valentine leuocidin-producing *Staphylococcus aureus* in primary skin infections and pneumonia. Clin Infect Dis 2003; 29:1128–1132.

17. Baggett H, Rudolph K, Hennessy T, et al. Panton-Valentine leukocidin (PVL) is associated with methicillin resistance in an outbreak of community-onset *Staphylococcus aureus* skin infections—Alaska. In: Program & Abstracts of the 40th Annual Infectious Disease Society of America meeting. Chicago, IL, 2002:126.

18. Schmitz FJ, MacKenzie CR, Geisel R, et al. Enterotoxin and toxic shock syndrome toxin-1 production of methicillin resistant and methicillin sensitive *Staphylococcus aureus* strains. Eur J Epidemiol 1997; 13:699–708.

19. Fujiwara Y, Endo S. A case of toxic shock syndrome secondary to mastitis caused by methicillin-resistant *Staphylococcus aureus*. Kansenshogaku Zasshi 2001; 75:898–903.

20. Amano T, Imao T, Fukuda M, Miwa S, Takemae K. Toxic shock syndrome due to methicillin resistant *Staphylococcus aureus* (MRSA) after total prostatectomy. Nippon Hinyokika Gakkai Zasshi 2002; 93:44–47.

21. Nakano M, Miyazawa H, Kawano Y, et al. An outbreak of neonatal toxic shock syndrome-like exanthematous disease (NTED) caused by methicillin-resistant *Staphylococcus aureus* (MRSA) in a neonatal intensive care unit. Microbiol Immunol 2002; 46:277–284.

22. Stevens DL, Herr D, Lampiris H, Hunt JL, Batts DH, Hafkin B, and the Linezolid MRSA Study Group. Linezolid versus vancomycin for the treatment of methicillin-resistant *Staphylococcus aureus* infections. Clin Infect Dis 2002; 34:1481–1490.

23. Jacobs MR, Amsler K, Bajaksouzian S, et al. Association between Panton Valentine leukociden and oxacillin resistance in *Staphylococcus aureus* in isolates from an international study of complicated skin and skin structure infections. ICCAC, Sept 2006 (poster K-0772).
24. Plouffe JF. Emerging therapies for serious gram-positive bacterial infections: a focus on linezolid. Clin Infect Dis 2000; 31(suppl 4):S144.
25. Conte J, Golden JA, Kipps J, Zurlinden E. Intrapulmonary pharmacokinetics of linezolid. Antimicrob Agents Chemo 2002; 46:1475–1480.
26. Fowler VG, Boucher HW, Corey R, et al. Daptomycin versus standard therapy for bacteremia and endocarditis caused by *Staphylococcus aureus*. New Engl J Med 2006; 355(7):653–665.
27. Gonzalez C, Rubio M, Romero-Vivas J, et al. Bacteremic pneumonia due to *Staphylococcus aureus*: a comparison of disease caused by methicillin-resistant and methicillin-susceptible organisms. Clin Infect Dis 1999; 29:1171.

Community-Acquired MRSA as a Pathogen

Karen J. Brasel and John A. Weigelt
Department of Surgery, Medical College of Wisconsin,
Milwaukee, Wisconsin, U.S.A.

DEFINITION

Community-acquired methicillin-resistant *Staphylococcus aureus* (CA-MRSA) was initially defined as an infection with methicillin-resistant *S. aureus* (MRSA) in an outpatient, or in a patient that manifested infection within 48 hours of hospital admission (1). However, it is now recognized that CA-MRSA has unique characteristics not related to time of onset or hospitalization that differentiate it from healthcare-associated MRSA (HA-MRSA). These include genetic profile, epidemiology, presentation, and treatment. Although there is no universally accepted definition, since 2000 the Centers for Disease Control definition of CA-MRSA is an infection with MRSA that lacks risk factors for a MRSA infection (Table 1) (2).

Current estimates of CA-MRSA prevalence vary from 5% to 49% (2,3). Such a wide range suggests that a single definition for CA-MRSA infection does not exist. A standard definition and subsequent case ascertainment is important to describe the epidemiology of this infection and to identify proper treatment principles.

BACTERIOLOGY

The hallmark of both CA-MRSA and HA-MRSA is methicillin and beta-lactam resistance, mediated by the altered penicillin binding protein 2a. The gene responsible for methicillin resistance, *mecA*, is located on a mobile chromosomal element called the staphylococcal cassette chromosome (SCC*mec*). There are five known types of the SCC.

TABLE 1 Centers for Disease Control Definition of MRSA

1. Isolation of MRSA more than 48 hours after hospital admission
2. History of hospitalization
3. Recent surgery
4. Dialysis
5. Residence in a long-term care facility
6. Presence of an indwelling catheter or a percutaneous
   device at the time of culture
7. Previous isolation of MRSA

Abbreviation: MRSA, methicillin-resistant *Staphylococcus aureus.*

Types I, II, and III, found in HA-MRSA, are relatively large and carry resistance to many different antibiotics. In contrast, CA-MRSA carries predominantly type IV (4,5). Type IV SCC was described in 2002 and is a much smaller SCC that lacks many of the other resistance genes common in HA-MRSA. SCC*mec* type V has recently been found in some strains of CA-MRSA from Australia (6).

SCC*mec* type IV was identified from isolates of *S. epidermidis* in the 1970s (7). Although CA-MRSA was described in an isolated outbreak in the late 1970s, widespread findings of CA-MRSA did not occur until 1989, suggesting that methicillin resistance may have originated in coagulase-negative bacteria. The small size of SCC*mec* type IV, in contrast to types II and III, likely contributes to the diversity of CA-MRSA strains as horizontal transfer of the small element is easily accomplished.

The Panton–Valentine leukocidin (PVL) gene is responsible for one of the most clinically significant virulence factors in CA-MRSA. The PVL gene, initially described in 1894 and further characterized by Panton and Valentine in 1932, encodes a pore-forming cytotoxin that acts preferentially against leukocytes and erythrocytes (8). It is commonly found in CA-MRSA infections and only rarely in HA-MRSA. In an epidemiologic study from Minnesota, it was present in 77% of all CA-MRSA and in only

4% of HA-MRSA (9). PVL toxin is found in almost all cases of furunculosis secondary to MRSA, the majority of cases of CA-MRSA pneumonia, approximately half of all cases of isolated cutaneous abscess and cellulitis, and a minority of cases of osteomyelitis (10,11). Although commonly found in CA-MRSA, the PVL gene is not genetically linked to SCC*mec* type IV. The PVL gene is found in methicillin-sensitive *S. aureus* and clearly predates the development of methicillin resistance, suggesting that CA-MRSA arose via transfer of SCC*mec* type IV into methicillin-sensitive strains of *S. aureus* with the PVL gene (12).

EPIDEMIOLOGY

The original outbreak of CA-MRSA was described in a population of intravenous drug users (13). The CA-MRSA infections were initially restricted to specific patient populations. Patients in closed populations predominated, including Native Americans, men who have sex with men, prison inmates, children in daycare centers, military recruits, and competitive athletes in team sports (11–14). However, the prevalence of CA-MRSA has increased to the point that many, if not the majority, of infections occur in patients without these risk factors. Infection and colonization has spread to include patients from Europe, Asia, Africa, South America, and Australia (10,11,14–17).

In the United States, the prevalence of MRSA in the general population was estimated from the 2001–2002 NHANES (National Health and Nutrition Examination Survey) data. The overall colonization rate of noninstitutionalized persons with methicillin-sensitive *S. aureus* is 31.6%, and 0.84% with MRSA. Prevalence rates in nonhospitalized patients around the world are similar; 0.7% in Portugal, 0.1% in Switzerland, and 0.03% in The Netherlands. Ten percent of the isolates resistant to methicillin obtained in the NHANES study underwent SCC*mec* typing to provide an estimate of the relative prevalence of HA-MRSA and CA-MRSA. Approximately half of those colonized with MRSA are colonized with SCC*mec* type II and half with SCC*mec* type

IV (18). The relative percentage of CA-MRSA colonization is higher than the relative percentage of CA-MRSA infections. On the basis of retrospective studies, the proportion of MRSA infections attributable to CA-MRSA is approximately 30%. In prospective series the incidence is somewhat higher at approximately 38% (1).

Risk factors associated with HA-MRSA infection ultimately guided recommendations for empiric MRSA treatment in high-risk hospitalized patients. The majority of these risk factors are not present in patients with CA-MRSA. In comparison to patients with infections due to HA-MRSA, those with CA-MRSA are younger and have tended to be in closed communities. Despite the clear differences between HA-MRSA and CA-MRSA, many patients with community-acquired infections have had recent contact with the healthcare system. This includes 62% who had visited a physician in the previous year, 39% who had received antimicrobial therapy, 33% with chronic noninfectious skin conditions, and 12% employed in a healthcare-related field within the previous five years (2,9).

Unfortunately, CA-MRSA has moved from closed communities with well-defined risk factors into the general population. It is almost endemic in many places. An explanation for this observation is transmission by asymptomatic carriers, who are colonized with CA-MRSA and form a large potential reservoir (18). Transmission from colonized healthcare workers has been described, most notably in outbreaks among healthy newborns whose mothers were not infected or colonized with MRSA (19). Transmission has also occurred between a healthy donor colonized with CA-MRSA to a liver transplant recipient, resulting in fatal necrotizing pneumonia (20). Mathematical modeling suggests that where it is not already endemic, a high likelihood exists that it will become so in the near future (21).

PRESENTATION

The majority of infections caused by CA-MRSA are skin and soft-tissue infections, accounting for approximately 75% of infections in adults and up to 90% of pediatric infections (9,22). The cytotoxicity conferred by the PVL gene results in an intense inflammatory cascade and extensive tissue necrosis. The resulting skin lesion can mimic a spider bite with central necrosis, surrounding induration and erythema (Fig. 1). This is particularly true in patients with no risk factors for an MRSA infection in areas where brown recluse spiders are endemic. As the six spider species that produce such a bite are geographically restricted (southern California, Arizona, and New Mexico; Texas, Oklahoma, Kansas, Iowa, Missouri, Illinois, Indiana, Ohio, Kentucky, Tennessee, Georgia, Alabama, Mississippi, Louisiana, and Arkansas), such lesions should be attributed to CA-MRSA in states outside this region. Even within endemic areas, given the increase in CA-MRSA, lesions are more likely due to CA-MRSA than spider bites (23). Lesions may be single or multiple, and satellite lesions are often

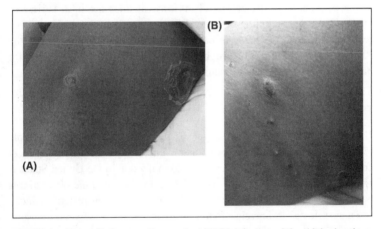

FIGURE 1 (**A** and **B**) Community-acquired MRSA infection of the thigh showing multiple lesions. A typical lesion has central necroses and surrounding induration, which is encircled by cellulitis.

present. Other skin and soft tissue manifestations include cellulitis and abscess.

Pneumonia is the second most common clinical manifestation of CA-MRSA. Many of these pneumonias are necrotizing, due to the presence of PVL gene. This results in mucosal ulcerations as well as hemorrhagic necrosis of the interalveolar septa. PVL-positive strains of *S. aureus* bind preferentially to damaged respiratory epithelium, explaining the association with prior influenza-like illnesses (24,25). In the 2003–2004 influenza season, 19 cases of CA-MRSA pneumonia were reported in the United States in patients with documented or suspected influenza preceding the MRSA infection. Fourteen of 15 isolates tested expressed the PVL toxin (25).

The potentially virulent nature of CA-MRSA infections was realized in the late 1990s, with the report of four fatalities in pediatric patients without previous risk factors (26). One patient suffered from a septic right hip, another meningitis, and two patients had pneumonia. Three patients were bacteremic at the time of their death. A variety of other infections, including osteomyelitis and meningitis, have now been reported due to CA-MRSA. In patients with pneumonia, presence of the PVL gene results in a much higher mortality, 37% compared to 6% for patients with PVL-negative pneumonia (10).

TREATMENT

Unlike HA-MRSA where the large SCC*mec* types I–III encode multiple resistance genes, SCC*mec* types IV and V encode relatively few. The most common strain of CA-MRSA causing skin infection in the United States is USA300-0114. USA300-0114 is resistant to four antimicrobial agents other than methicillin and penicillin. The most common pattern included resistance to erythromycin, found in over 90%. A separate plasmid encodes for tetracycline resistance, which occurred in 23% of isolates. Inducible resistance to levofloxacin was present in 20%. Clindamycin resistance, which can be either inducible or constitutive, is encoded by another plasmid and was present in 13%. The combination of resistance to all four additional antimicrobial agents was not described (27). Resistance patterns differ notably by geographic region, with clindamycin resistance more prevalent in the southern United States (27,28).

No studies of various treatment regimens are available to guide treatment of patients with a CA-MRSA infection. A variety of oral agents are available to treat mild to moderate infections with CA-MRSA based on resistance patterns for the bacteria. Trimethoprim-sulfamethoxazole and doxycycline are both acceptable, as the resistance rates to both of these agents are low. Neither agent has activity against streptococci—potentially problematic in treating cellulitis or other infections where the causative gram-positive agent may not be known. Clindamycin has broader activity against gram-positive infections, but must be used with some caution due to the potential for inducible resistance. Inducible resistance is not found in strains that are susceptible to erythromycin; however, the majority of strains responsible for soft-tissue infections are erythromycin-resistant. Inducible clindamycin resistance can be detected by using the double disk diffusion test (D test). This test was recommended as the standard by the Clinical and Laboratory Standards Institute (CLSI, formerly NCCLS) in 2004 and is now routine in many laboratories, but can delay results of susceptibility testing by 24 to 48 hours (28).

Severe or invasive infections due to CA-MRSA require hospitalization and intravenous antibiotics. Intravenous forms of the aforementioned antimicrobials are effective for these infections, although should only be used if HA-MRSA is not a concern. If HA-MRSA is a possibility, vancomycin, daptomycin, linezolid, tigecycline, or quinupristin-dalfopristin (not Food and Drug Administration-approved for MRSA) should be used until results of sensitivity testing are available. Whether agents that shut down toxin production, such as clindamycin, tetracycline, and linezolid, are specifically more effective in PVL-positive strains of CA-MRSA infection is unknown. Linezolid is more effective than vancomycin in treating both pneumonia and complicated skin and soft-tissue infections due to the combination of CA-MRSA and HA-MRSA (29). It is unclear whether this will remain true for pneumonia and soft tissue infections due solely to CA-MRSA.

Resistance patterns, in addition to varying by geographic region, also vary by age. In a group of patients treated at the University of Chicago, erythromycin, clindamycin, ciprofloxacin, gentamicin, and tetracycline resistance was much more common in adult patients than pediatric patients. Particularly striking was the difference in resistance to clindamycin: 52% in adults compared to 7% in pediatric patients (30). This has led to the use of clindamycin as a first-line agent in many CA-MRSA infections in the pediatric population.

A hallmark of CA-MRSA infections is inadequate initial antibiotic therapy (9). This occurs because the majority of patients with CA-MRSA infections do not have risk factors to trigger the clinician's concern for a possible MRSA infection. Knowledge of endemic rates of CA-MRSA, careful assessment of potential risk factors, and recognition of lesions typical of CA-MRSA are all necessary to ensure adequacy of initial treatment. In our experience, CA-MRSA should be suspected in any patient with a skin lesion that has central necrosis, surrounding erythema and a large amount of induration. Satellite lesions should increase suspicion for a CA-MRSA infection.

Surgical treatment has been the standard treatment for soft-tissue abscesses, including those due to CA-MRSA and HA-MRSA. Incision and drainage is recommended, with concomitant antibiotic therapy indicated for surrounding cellulitis or systemic illness. Perhaps because of the presence of the PVL gene in many of these infections, small abscesses contain a minimal amount of drainable material; the majority of the infection or "abscess" is an intense inflammatory reaction. Rather than multiple incisions that yield minimal results, the authors had good success in treating adult patients with oral antibiotics and close follow-up. The typical course is a lesion that dries up over the course of five to seven days. A patient is usually treated for five days and re-evaluated. Longer courses are rarely needed despite the 10- to 12-day duration reported in the largest MRSA complicated skin and skin structure study

(29). Treatment failures after five to seven days may need surgical drainage, but in the authors' experience these have been the minority of cases. Treatment failures may be secondary to drug resistance and if no improvement occurs after five days, then use of a HA-MRSA drug is the authors' approach. Oral therapy is commonly continued with linezolid in patients who fail initial therapy with either doxycycline or clindamycin. Hospitalization is rarely indicated if the correct diagnosis is made and the patient has no systemic signs of toxicity.

PREVENTION

Standard infection control principles are the best method to prevent outbreaks due to CA-MRSA. These include hand washing, daily showers, use of antibacterial soap, covering any draining lesions, isolation of infected patients needing hospitalization, and avoidance of sharing personal items. Isolation may require withholding athletes with draining wounds from competition, and not allowing healthcare workers with open wounds to return to work until they have healed (14). Contact isolation procedures should be used for hospitalized patients.

Immunization has been attempted in high risk dialysis patients (31). Partial immunity was achieved, but it did not last. No vaccine is approved for clinical use at this time. Decolonization has been attempted both for outbreak control and to prevent recurrence. Various strategies, including systemic antibiotics, chlorhexidine body washes, and mupiricin nasal ointment, have been tried with limited effectiveness. Although there are insufficient data to recommend any one strategy over another, decolonization is probably worthwhile in high-risk patient populations and with recurrent disease in an individual or in families (14,32).

CONCLUSIONS

CA-MRSA is clearly different from HA-MRSA. Although the population prevalence of asymptomatic colonization in the United States is relatively low, it will only increase. The proportion of Staphylococcal infections due to CA-MRSA has reached the point where empiric coverage against this pathogen should be considered in many cases. Recognition of typical skin lesions, pneumonia associated with influenza-like illnesses, and identification of historical risk factors will help institute appropriate therapy early.

REFERENCES

1. Salgado CD, Farr BM, Calfee DP. Community-acquired methicillin-resistant *Staphylococcus aureus*: a meta-analysis of prevalence and risk factors. Clin Infect Dis 2003; 36:131–139.
2. Fridkin SK, Hageman JC, Morrison M, et al. Methicillin-resistant *Staphylococcus aureus* disease in three communities. N Engl J Med 2005; 352:1436–1444.
3. Folden DV, Machayya JA, Sahmoun AE, et al. Estimating the proportion of community-associated methicillin-resistant *Staphylococcus aureus*: two definitions used in the USA yield dramatically different estimates. J Hosp Infect 2005; 60:329–332.
4. Tenover FC, McDougal LK, Goering RV. Characterization of a strain of community-associated methicillin-resistant *Staphylococcus aureus* widely disseminated in the United States. J Clin Micro 2006; 44:108–118.
5. Ma XX, Ito T, Tiensasitorn C, et al. Novel type of staphylococcal cassette chromosome mec identified in community-acquired methicillin-resistant *Staphylococcus aureus* strains. Antimicrob Agents Chemother 2002; 46:1147–1152.
6. O'Brien FG, Coombs GW, Pearson JC, et al. Type V staphylococcal cassette chromosome *mec* in community staphylococci from Australia. Antimicrob Agents Chemother 2005; 49:5129–5132.
7. Wisplinghoff H, Rosato AE, Enright MC, et al. Related clones containing SCCmec type IV predominate among clinically significant *Staphylococcus epidermidis* isolates. Antimicrob Agents Chemother 2003; 47:3574–3579.
8. Panton PN, Valentine FCO. Staphylococcal toxin. Lancet 1932; 1:506–508.
9. Naimi TS, LeDell KN, Como-Sabetti K, et al. Comparison of community- and health care-associated methicillin-resistant *Staphylococcus aureus* infection. J Am Med Assoc 2003; 290:2976–2984.
10. Kollef MH, Micek ST. Methicillin-resistant *Staphylococcus aureus*: a new community-acquired pathogen? Curr Opinion Infect Dis 2006; 19:161–168.

11. Gosbell IB. Epidemiology, clinical features and management of infections due to community methicillin-resistant *Staphylococcus aureus* (cMRSA). Int Med J 2005; 35:S120–S135.

12. Nolte O, Haag H, Zimmerman A, Geiss HK. *Staphylococcus aureus* positive for Panton-Valentine leukocidin genes but susceptible to methicillin in patients with furuncles. Eur J Clin Microbiol Infect Dis 2005; 24:477–479.

13. Saravolatz LD, Markowitz N, Arking L, et al. Epidemiologic observations during a community-acquired outbreak. Ann Intern Med 1982; 96:11–16.

14. Kowalski TJ, Berbari EF, Osmon DR. Epidemiology, treatment, and prevention of community-acquired methicillin-resistant *Staphylococcus aureus* infections. Mayo Clin Proc 2005; 80:1201–1208.

15. von Specht M, Gardella N, Tagliaferri P, et al. Methicillin-resistant *Staphylococcus aureus* in community-acquired meningitis. Eur J Clin Microbiol Infect Dis 2006; 25:267–269.

16. Naas T, Fortineau N, Spicq C, et al. Three-year survey of community-acquired methicillin-resistant *Staphylococcus aureus* producing Panton-Valentine leukocidin in a French university hospital. J Hosp Infect 2006; 61:321–329.

17. Kluytmans-VendenBergh MFQ, Kluytmans JAJW. Community-acquired methicillin-resistant *Staphylococcus aureus*: current perspectives. Clin Micro Infect 2006; 12:9–15.

18. Graham PL, Lin SX, Larson EL. A U.S. population-based survey of *Staphylococcus aureus* colonization. Ann Intern Med 2006; 144:318–325.

19. MMWR 2006; 55:329–332.

20. Obed A, Schnitzbauer AA, Bein T, et al. Fatal pneumonia caused by Panton-Valentine leukocidin-positive methicillin-resistant *Staphylococcus aureus* transmitted from a healthy donor in living-donor liver transplantation. Transplantation 2006; 81:121–124.

21. Cooper BS, Medley GF, Stone SP, et al. Methicillin-resistant *Staphylococcus aureus* in hospitals and the community: stealth dynamics and control catastrophes. Proc Natl Acad Sci USA 2004; 101:10,223–10,228.

22. Kaplan SL. Implications of methicillin-resistant *Staphylococcus aureus* as a community-acquired pathogen in pediatric patients. Infect Dis Clin N Am 2005; 19:747–757.

23. Swanson DL, Vetter RS. Bites of brown recluse spiders and suspected necrotic arachnidism. N Engl J Med 2005; 352:700–707.

24. Francis JS, Doherty MC, Lopatin U, et al. Severe community-onset pneumonia in healthy adults caused by methicillin-resistant *Staphylococcus aureus* carrying the Panton-Valentine leukocidin genes. Clin infect Dis 2005; 40:100–107.

25. Hageman JC, Uyeki TM, Francis JS, et al. Severe community-acquired pneumonia due to *Staphylococcus aureus*, 2003–2004 influenza season. Emerg Infect Dis 2006; 12:894–899.

26. MMWR 1999;48:707–710.

27. King MD, Humphrey BJ, Wang YF, et al. Emergence of community-acquired methicillin-resistant *Staphylococcus aureus* USA 300 clone as the predominant cause of skin and soft-tissue infections. Ann Intern Med 2006; 144:309–317.

28. Lewis JS, Jorgensen JH. Inducible clindamycin resistance in staphylococci: should clinicians and microbiologists be concerned? Clin Infect Dis 2005; 40:280–285.

29. Weigelt JA, Itani K, Stevens D, et al. Linezolid versus vancomycin in treatment of complicated skin and soft tissue infections. Antimicrob Agents Chemother 2005; 49:2260–2266.

30. David MZ, Crawford SE, Boyle-Vavra S, et al. Contrasting pediatric and acult methicillin-resistant *Staphylococcus aureus* isolates. Emerg Infect Dis 2006; 12:631–637.

31. Shinefield H, Black S, Fattom A, et al. Use of a *Staphylococcus aureus* conjugate vaccine in patients receiving hemodialysis. N Engl J Med 2002; 346:491–496.

32. Khoury J, Jones M, Grim A, et al. Eradication of methicillin-resistant *Staphylococcus aureus* from a neonatal intensive care unit by active surveillance and aggressive infection control measures. Infect Cont Hosp Ep 2005; 26:616–621.

MRSA and Complicated Skin and Soft Tissue Infections

5

Kamal M. F. Itani
Department of Surgery, Boston Veterans Affairs Health Care System,
Boston University, Boston, Massachusetts, U.S.A.

DEFINITION

Infections involving skin and soft tissue are referred to by two synonymous terms: skin and skin structure infections and skin and soft tissue infections (SSTIs), complicated or uncomplicated (1). Uncomplicated SSTI include superficial infections, such as cellulitis, simple abscesses, impetigo, and furuncles. In most instances, these infections can be treated by surgical incision alone or in the case of cellulitis with antibiotics alone.

The complicated SSTI (cSSTI) category includes infections either involving deeper soft tissue or requiring significant surgical intervention, such as infected ulcers, burns and major abscesses or a significant underlying disease state and comorbidities that complicate the response to treatment. Superficial infections or abscesses in an anatomical site, such as the rectal area, where the risk of anaerobic or gram-negative pathogen involvement is higher, should be considered complicated infections (1). SSTIs in critical anatomical locations such as the face and periorbital areas as well as the neck, hands, and feet should be also considered complicated.

For uncomplicated SSTI, the two most common pathogens are *Staphylococcus aureus* and *Streptococcus pyogenes*. Other isolated organisms are not uniformly considered pathogens in this condition, but rather seen as colonizers or contaminants. For cSSTI, the possible pathogens are numerous and dependent on the clinical situation, the location of the lesion/infection, and past medical history of the patient. In addition, it is sometimes difficult to separate a colonizer from a pathogen, since the same organism can be either one, depending on the clinical setting (1).

There is a continuum from contamination to colonization and finally infection. Contamination has no signs of local or systemic response. As the wound becomes progressively colonized with rising bacterial counts, subtle local signs occur signaling a change in the equilibrium or an increasing bioburden contributing to abnormal wound homeostasis, and possible delayed healing. Infection occurs when the bacteria have invaded the tissue, are multiplying, and cause a systemic host reaction and impaired healing. While infection in acute wounds may be easy to identify, the chronic colonized wound often presents a challenge when trying to identify signs and symptoms of infection.

Staphylococcal cSSTI can be caused by methicillin-sensitive *S. aureus* (MSSA) or methicillin-resistant *S. aureus* (MRSA) bacteria. A recent increase in prevalence of MRSA cSSTI has caused a re-evaluation of treatment principles.

COMMUNITY-ACQUIRED AND HEALTHCARE-RELATED MRSA IN SKIN AND SOFT TISSUE INFECTIONS

Until recently, drug-resistant strains of *S. aureus* were considered to be acquired almost exclusively in hospital settings, but reports of MRSA acquired in the community are increasing, and are most often associated with SSTI. In the SENTRY antimicrobial surveillance program, *S. aureus* was found to be the predominant pathogen in nosocomial SSTI accounting for 45.9% of isolates. Thirty percent of *S. aureus* isolates were methicillin resistant (2).

In a prospective cohort study of MRSA cases conducted in Minnesota in the year 2000, 12% of the strains were community-acquired MRSA (CA-MRSA), accounting for 75% of all SSTI in that population (3). Although CA-MRSA is usually resistant to the beta-lactam group of antibiotics, it is usually susceptible in vitro to fluoroquinolones, trimethoprim/sulfamethoxazole, clindamycin, and chloramphenicol. This is in contradistinction to healthcare-acquired MRSA (HA-MRSA), which is usually resistant to fluoroquinolones, clindamycin, and chloremphenicol, and is less sensitive to trimethoprim/sulfamethoxazole. Clusters of CA-MRSA cSSTI have been documented among athletes participating in contact sports, military recruits, Pacific Islanders, Alaskan natives, Native Americans, men who have sex with men, IV drug users, and prisoners (4). Correctional inmates with HIV infections are twice as likely to develop MRSA infections compared with HIV-negative inmates (4). Factors associated with the spread of CA-MRSA skin infections in otherwise healthy people include close skin-to-skin contact, openings in the skin such as cuts or abrasions, contaminated items and surfaces, crowded living conditions, and poor hygiene. In a case-controlled study, persons with CA-MRSA SSTI had received significantly more courses of antibiotics in the year before the outbreak (a median of 4 vs. 2 courses, $P = 0.01$) (5).

Risk factors for HA-MRSA infection include a current or recent hospitalization, residing in a long-term care facility, previous infection with MRSA, chronic wounds, and patients with invasive devices, such as dialysis, Foley catheters, feeding tubes, and intravenous catheters.

SIGNS AND SYMPTOMS

Infections with *S. aureus*, including MRSA, generally start as small, red bumps that resemble pimples. They can become deep, painful abscesses that require surgical drainage. Most of the time, the bacteria remain confined to the skin, but they can cause potentially life-threatening infections in bones, joints, surgical wounds, the bloodstream, heart valves, and lungs. Unlike HA-MRSA, CA-MRSA produces the Panton–Valentine leukocidin toxin that destroys white blood cells and living tissue. The toxin can cause severe, often fatal skin infections (necrotizing fasciitis) and pneumonia.

Necrotizing Skin and Soft Tissue Infection
Necrotizing fasciitis is a rapidly progressive, life-threatening infection involving the skin, soft tissue, and deep fascia. These infections are

typically caused by a group A *Streptococcus*, *Clostridium perfringens*, or a mixture of aerobic and anaerobic organisms, typically including group A streptococcus, the enterobacteriacae, and anaerobes. In the past, *S. aureus* has been a very uncommon cause of necrotizing fasciitis, but CA-MRSA is an emerging cause of necrotizing fasciitis (6). In a recent report of 14 patients with MRSA necrotizing fasciitis, necrotizing myositis, or both, the median age was 46 years and 71% were men. Coexisting or risk factors included current or past infection, drug use (43%), previous MRSA infection, diabetes, and chronic hepatitis C (21% each). Wound cultures were monomicrobial for MRSA in 86% of cases. All MRSA isolates were susceptible in vitro to clindamycin, trimethoprim/sulfamethoxazole, and rifampin. All recovered isolates were mec type IV and carried the Panton–Valentine leukocidin gene. The author suggests that in areas where CA-MRSA infections are endemic, empirical therapy for MRSA infection should not be withheld from patients with suspected necrotizing fascitis on the basis of the absence of clinical risk factors. This is a distinct change in the approach to the patient with a necrotizing skin and soft tissue infection, as therapy against CA-MRSA is not currently recommended for these patients (6).

Surgical Site Infection

Infections of surgical wounds are the most common adverse events affecting hospitalized patients who have undergone surgery. Recent data from the Centers for Disease Control show a 2.6% incidence of surgical site infections (SSIs), although this incidence is believed to be higher due to inadequate post discharge surveillance (7). The frequency of SSI is related to the category of operation, with clean and low-risk operations having the lowest rate of infection and contamination and high-risk operations having greater infection rates. Scoring system have been developed to predict the risk of SSI, the most popular of which is the one developed by the National Nosocomial Infection Surveillance (NNIS) (8). Data for the NNIS system were derived from 44 participating hospitals and conducted by the CDC. Traditional wound class of contaminated or dirty/infected was maintained as one of the factors used to predict risk for wound infection. The American Society of Anesthesiologists (ASA) physical status classification replaced the number of discharge diagnoses as the second factor. An ASA score of 3 or greater garners one point in the NNIS system. Duration of the operation is the third factor, and is worth one point if the procedure lasts longer than 75% of similar procedures. A patient's risk for surgical site infection can therefore be stratified as NNIS class 0, 1, 2, or 3, based on which of the three risk factors the patient has. Although the risk of infection increases within the wound classification, it has been shown to be also dependent within each wound class on the NNIS classification (Table 1) (9).

The type of organism encountered in a SSI depends on the type of surgery performed; gram-positive organisms are more likely to be encountered in clean cases, whereas gram-negative organisms are more likely to be encountered in clean contaminated cases involving the alimentary tract. The most prevalent pathogen isolated from SSIs is *S. aureus*. The prevalence of *S. aureus* as a pathogen in surgical infections has remained constant, whereas the proportion of isolates identified as MRSA has continued to increase. According to reports from the SENTRY Antimicrobial

TABLE 1 Surgical Site Infection Rates by Wound Class versus National Nosocomical Infection Surveillance Class

Wound class	All (%)	NNIS 0 (%)	NNIS 1 (%)	NNIS 2 (%)	NNIS 3 (%)
Clean	2.1	1.0	2.3	5.4	N/A
Clean contaminated	3.3	2.1	4.0	9.5	N/A
Contaminated	6.4	N/A	3.4	6.8	13.2
Dirty/infected	7.1	N/A	3.1	8.1	12.8
All	2.8	1.5	2.9	6.8	13.0

Source: From Ref. 9.

Surveillance Program from the United States and Canada in 2000, MRSA is responsible for 30% of SSIs compared to 24% three years earlier (10,11). Increased rates of MRSA infections are of particular concern because patients infected with this pathogen have higher mortality rates, greater morbidity, and utilize more healthcare resources compared with those who have infections caused by methicillin-susceptible pathogens (12,13).

Successful therapy of these infections depends on the early suspicion and identification of resistant pathogens and subsequent use of antibiotics against MRSA.

Prophylaxis for surgical site infection is a well-established practice and the target of performance improvement in the United States. Surgical site prophylaxis for many clean surgical cases uses drugs that have been effective against MSSA. The explosion of MRSA, whether it is CA-MRSA or HA-MRSA, has produced a dilemma. Prophylaxis for MRSA SSI remains a source of controversy; however, as delineated by the CDC, patients at a high risk for MRSA should undergo prophylaxis with an anti-MRSA agent (14). Mupirocin treatment of *S. aureus* colonized patients prior to surgery has not been shown to decrease the incidence of surgical site infection (15). No guidelines exist about the decolonization of patients prior to surgery; as part of infection control measures, decolonization of patients detected to be MRSA colonized has been practiced in certain hospitals (16).

Blistering Distal Dactylitis

Blistering distal dactylis (BDD) is a distinct clinical entity involving localized infection of the volar fat pad of the distal phalynx of the fingers and sometimes toes. If left untreated, it can lead to progression and distal digit amputation. It should be differentiated from bullous impetigo, which has the same etiology but is more superficial (Fig. 1).

The characteristic clinical appearance is fluid-filled blisters containing thin, white pus. The BDD is typically seen in children between the ages of 2 and 16 years, although it has also been reported in infants and adults.

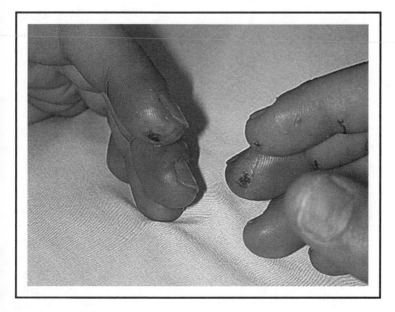

FIGURE 1   Blistering distal dactylitis. *Source*: From Ref. 17.

Autoinoculation of the finger from nose picking is one proposed course. The BDD is usually associated with group A beta-hemolytic streptococcus, but can also be caused by *S. aureus* and *S. epidermidis*. Multiple finger involvement may be a predictor of *S. aureus* infection. Increasing reports of MRSA BDD is being reported, necessitating appropriate antibiotic coverage for this organism (17).

MANAGEMENT OF COMPLICATED SKIN AND SOFT TISSUE INFECTIONS

The management of cSSTI is based on two important considerations: (*i*) the host risk factors and (*ii*) the systemic host response to the infection.

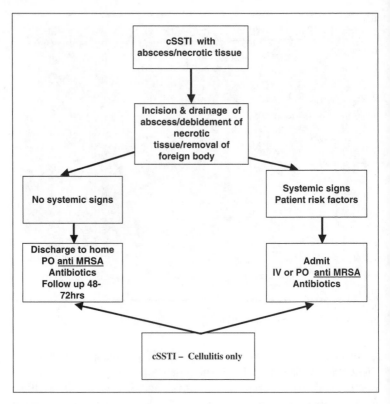

FIGURE 2 Management of MRSA-complicated skin and soft tissue infections.

On the basis of these two considerations, a management algorithm was developed and is shown in Figure 2.

The host risk factors well established for SSI are multiple and include increasing age, poor nutritional status, uncontrolled diabetes, impaired immunity, obesity, and poor tissue oxygenation at the site of incision. Less important risk factors include nicotine use, prior hospitalization, and other infections at a remote site from the site in question. In addition to environmental factors in the operating room and surgical technique, these lesser factors are important risk factors for surgical site infection and other cSSTI (18).

Systemic host response is manifested by increasing temperature and WBC; great caution needs to be applied in the elderly, the very young, and the immunocompromised, as the systemic responses could be attenuated, manifesting only as a low grade temperature, hypothermia, a left shift, leucopenia, systemic sepsis, or local symptoms only.

Surgical intervention is the mainstay of therapy, consisting of incision and drainage of abscesses and debridement of all necrotic tissue, and removal of any foreign bodies. The only exception is cellulitis. Caution has to be exercised with cellulitis. Cellulitis may be appropriately treated with antibiotics alone, but unresolving cellulitis with appropriate antibiotic therapy should prompt an evaluation for a deep abscess or underlying fascitis. Removal of foreign bodies, including suture material, artificial mesh, and prosthetics, is important. Foreign bodies serve as a nidus for bacteria and are associated with biofilm formation and bacterial deposition, which facilitates persistence of infection. The biofilm around the foreign body also prevents antibiotics from reaching the bacteria.

Antibiotic therapy is usually an adjuvant to surgical therapy. In patients with MRSA risk factors, systemic manifestations or deep tissue infections, antibiotics should be administered. Whether antibiotics are given orally or intravenously is dependent on the extent of infection, presence or absence of systemic symptoms, and the availability of an oral antibiotic that will effectively cover suspected or proven organisms (Fig. 2). Hospitalization is usually determined by the patient's overall clinical status and whether the patient needs intravenous antibiotics. Arrangements can also be made for intravenous antibiotics to be administered at home if no oral counterpart is available and the patient's clinical status permits.

Poor response to therapy manifesting as persistence of local or systemic symptoms imply inadequate source control, poor drainage of an abscess, or resistance of the bacteria to chosen antibiotics. Debridement of remaining or new necrotic tissue should be performed; a search for undrained abscesses should be performed with ultrasonography or computed tomography. Osteomyelitis should be suspected in patients with diabetic foot infections. If the site of infection is clean and no other source is located, appropriate tissue cultures should be obtained, and when MRSA is suspected another antibiotic with MRSA activity should be tried.

The length of antibiotic therapy in cSSTI has not been addressed. It is my belief that the duration of antibiotic therapy is dependent on resolution of local and systemic symptoms rather than on a specific number of days. In young, healthy individuals, antibiotics can be stopped as soon as local and systemic symptoms have resolved. This should also be considered in patients with risk factors, although greater caution should be exercised, especially if the host is immunocompromised. Antibiotics should be used for longer periods in patients with diabetic foot infections and patients with osteomyelitis. The duration of treatment remains controversial and is dependent on the extent of bone debridement, extent of vascular disease, and local improvement of local signs (19).

CHOICE OF ANTIBIOTICS IN MRSA-COMPLICATED SKIN AND SOFT TISSUE INFECTION

Because MRSA infection rates continue to increase, both in the hospital and the community, resistance needs to be considered when designing a treatment regimen for cSSTI. Factors that determine success or failure of an antimicrobial agent in treating a specific infection include the site of infection and the spectrum of activity, efficacy, and safety profile (20). Both patient factors and prevalence of MRSA influence the choice of empirical antibiotics. Individual risk factors need to be considered, in addition to the prevalence of MRSA within a particular institution or population group. Some facilities use a tool to predict the probability of methicillin resistance in patients with a suspected *S. aureus* infection

(21,22). If CA-MRSA is strongly suspected on the basis of local prevalence data or epidemiological and/or clinical clues, coverage for that organism becomes essential. Appropriate outpatient treatment can be given with trimethoprim-sulfamethoxazole (TMP-SMX), minocycline, doxycycline, or clindamycin. Numerous treatment failures have been attributed to inducible clindamycin resistance: any erythromycin-resistant but clindamycin-susceptible strain may harbor inducible resistance (23). None of these drugs is FDA-approved for MRSA cSSTI, and none have undergone rigorous evaluation in clinical trials. In addition, no randomized prospective data are available to support one oral agent over another in this setting. However, the availability, low cost, and long-standing use of these drugs in clinical practice have given them a de-facto acceptance for the treatment of MRSA cSSTI.

Newer fluoroquinolones (e.g., gatifloxacin, moxifloxacin, and levofloxacin) have enhanced activity against *Staphylococcus*, and combined with rifampin, appear effective in diverse clinical scenarios (24). Increasing fluoroquinolone resistance among CA-MRSA, some of the gram-negative bacilli and the association of fluoroquinolones with clostridium difficile colitis suggest that fluoroquinolones should not be first-line agents for empirical treatment (25).

Several other antimicrobials are available for the treatment of MRSA cSSTI. Vancomycin has been the treatment of choice for infections caused by MRSA; however, current data indicate that it may not be the optimal choice in cSSTI. Thirty years after vancomycin became available, vancomycin-resistant Enterococci (VRE) was first identified in France in 1986. Of great concern was the emergence of reduced vancomycin susceptibility in *S. aureus*, which many feared to be a prelude to full resistance. Since 1996, vancomycin-intermediate-resistant *S. aureus* (VISA) has been identified in Europe, Asia, and the United States. Rare strains demonstrating complete resistance to vancomycin have emerged and are known as vancomycin-resistant *S. aureus* (VRSA). As a result of this developing resistance, several new antimicrobials against MRSA have received FDA approval for treating MRSA cSSTI. Linezolid, daptomycin, and tigecycline have been approved for use in MRSA cSSTI; quinupristin/dalfopristin was approved for cSSTI but not cSSTI due to MRSA.

A large prospective, randomized, multinational trial compared linezolid to vancomycin or a semisynthetic penicillin in 1200 patients with cSSTI. Clinical cure was achieved in 92.2% and 88.5% of patients treated with linezolid and vancomycin, respectively ($P = 0.057$). A total of 134 patients with MRSA cSSTI were found in both the linezolid and vancomycin group. Patient outcome with MRSA infections was better when treated with linezolid; 88.6% cure versus 66.9% cure for patients treated with vancomycin ($P < 0.001$) (26). A subset analysis from this trial compared 66 patients with SSI receiving linezolid to 69 SSI patients receiving vancomycin for clinical and microbiologic cure. Among patients with MRSA infections, clinical cure in both groups was similar, but microbiologic eradication of the bacteria from the wound was achieved in 87% of the SSI patients treated with linezolid versus 48% treated with vancomycin ($P = 0.0022$) (27). Linezolid is the only agent with available pharmacoeconomic data. Though it has a high acquisition cost, it is 100% bioavailable when administered orally, and markedly reduces the length of intravenous therapy. Reduction in intravenous therapy was almost 11 days in patients with MRSA infections (1.8 days on linezolid to 12.6 days on vancomycin), and by seven days overall. Length of stay was decreased by at least two days when infections caused by methicillin-sensitive or methicillin-resistant organisms were treated with linezolid (28). Incremental analysis of total costs and cure showed that linezolid resulted in a mean 5.7% increase in clinical cure rate concomitant with a mean $652 in cost saving per patient treated for cSSTI in the intent to treat population (29).

Daptomycin was compared with vancomycin or semisynthetic penicillin in a phase 3, multicenter, double blind study consisting of 562 patients with cSSTI. Clinical cure of 81% was observed in both groups. Microbiologic eradication was achieved in 91% of patients treated with daptomycin versus 92% of patients treated with comparators (30).

Tigecycline is a novel glycopeptide that displays expanded broad-spectrum activity against gram-positive cocci, including MRSA and VRE, gram-negative bacilli, atypical organisms and anaerobes. Clinical trials of tigecycline for cSSTI have demonstrated equivalent efficacy to vancomycin and suggest that it will be a reasonable alternative for multidrug-resistant organisms (31). The broad-spectrum activity of tigecycline makes it an agent for consideration in patients with cSSTI secondary to multiple organisms often seen in patients with perirectal abscesses and necrotizing fasciitis.

Several novel antimicrobials with activity against MRSA cSSTI are currently awaiting FDA clearance or in late phase 3 trials and include dalbavancin, oritavancin, and theravance. Longer half-lives with more convenient dosing schedules is one possible advantage of these newer agents.

The choice of any of these newer FDA-approved agents as opposed to the older agents that show activity against CA-MRSA is not easy. The clinician must consider the likelihood of CA-MRSA versus HA-MRSA, patient drug allergies, drug interactions, pharmacokinetics, available oral therapy for outpatient use, pharmacoeconomic data and the emergence resistant organisms in the future with widespread utilization.

REFERENCES

1. Uncomplicated and complicated skin and skin structure infections—developing Antimicrobial drugs for treatment: Guidance for Industry. www.fda.gov/cder/guidance/2566dfr.pdf 7-22-1998. Last accessed August 12, 2006.
2. Rennie RP, Jones RN, Mutnick AH; SENTRY Program Study Group (North America). Occurrence and antimicrobial susceptibility patterns of pathogens isolated from skin and soft tissue infections: report from the SENTRY Antimicrobial Surveillance Program (United States and Canada, 2000). Diagn Microbiol Infect Dis 2003; 45(4):287–293.
3. Naimi TS, LeDell KH, Como-Sabetti K, et al. Comparison of community- and health care-associated methicillin-resistant *Staphylococcus aureus* infection. J Am Med Assoc 2003; 290(22):2976–2984.

4. Weber JT. Community-associated methicillin-resistant *Staphylococcus aureus*. Clin Infect Dis 2005; 41(suppl 4):S269–S272.
5. Baggett HC, Hennessy TW, Rudolph K, et al. Community-onset methicillin-resistant *Staphylococcus aureus* associated with antibiotic use and the cytotoxin Panton-Valentine leukocidin during a furunculosis outbreak in rural Alaska. J Infect Dis 2004; 189(9):1565–1573.
6. Miller LG, Perdreau-Remmington F, Rieg G, et al. Necrotizing fasciitis caused by community-associated methicillin-resistant *Staplylococcus aureus* in Los Angeles. N Engl J Med 2005; 352:1445–1453.
7. Horan TC, Gaynes RP, Martone WJ, et al. CDC definitions of nosocomial surgical site infections. Infect Control Hosp Epidemiol 1992; 13:606–608.
8. Culver DH, Horan TC, Gaynes RP, et al. Surgical wound infection rates by wound class, operative procedure, and patient risk index. Am J Med 1991; 91 (suppl 3B):152–157.
9. Knight R, Charbonneau P, Ratzer E, et al. Prophylactic antibiotics are not indicated in clean general surgery cases. Am J Surg 2001; 182:682–686.
10. Rennie RP, Jones RN, Mutnick AH; SENTRY Study Group (North America). Occurrence and antimicrobial susceptibility patterns of pathogens isolated from skin and soft tissue infection: report from the SENTRY Antimicrobial Surveillance Program (United States and Canada, 2000). Diagn Microbial Infect Dis 2003; 45:287–293.
11. Doern GV, Jones RN, Pfaller MA, et al. and the SENTRY study group (North America). Bacterial pathogens isolated from patients with skin and soft tissue infections: frequency of occurrence and antimicrobial susceptibility patterns from the SENTRY Antimicrobial Surveillance Program (United States and Canada, 1997). Diagn Microbiol Infect Dis 1999; 34:65–72.
12. Kaye KS, Engemann JJ, Mozaffari E, Carmeli Y. Reference group choice and antibiotic resistance outcomes. Emerg Infect Dis 2004; 10(6):1125–1128.
13. Engemann JJ, Carmeli Y, Cosgrove SE, et al. Adverse clinical and economic outcomes attributable to methicillin resistance among patients with *Staphylococcus aureus* surgical site infection. Clin Infect Dis 2003; 36(5):592–598.
14. Bratzler DW, Houck PM; Surgical Infection Prevention Guidelines Writers Workgroup. Antimicrobial prophylaxis for surgery: an advisory statement from the National Surgical Infection Prevention Project. Clin Infect Dis 2004; 38(12):1706.
15. Perl TM, Cullen JJ, Wenzel RP, Zimmerman MB, et al. Intranasal mupirocin to prevent postoperative *Staphylococcus aureus* infection. N Engl J Med 2002 Jun 13; 346(24):1871–1877.

16. Rao N, Jacobs S, Joyce L. Cost-effective eradication of an outbreak of methicillin-resistant *Staphylococcus aureus* in a community teaching hospital. Infect Control Hosp Epidemiol 1988 Jun; 9(6):255–260.

17. Huh SY, Daya M. Dermatology quiz. Resident and staff physician 2006; 852(6):37–38.

18. Mangram AJ, Horan TC, Pearson ML, Silver LC, Jarvis, WR. Guideline for prevention of surgical site infection, 1999. Hospital Infection Control Practices Advisory Committee. Infec Control Hosp Epidemiol 1999; 20(4):250–278.

19. Lipsky BA, Berendt AR, Deery HG, et al. Diagnosis and treatment of diabetic foot infections. Clin Infect Dis 2004; 39(7):885–910.

20. Stevens DL. The relevance of antibiotic tissue penetration for treating complicated skin and soft tissue infections caused by methicillin-resistant *Staphylococcus aureus*: an evidence-based review. Med Ed Direct 2004; 4:1–6.

21. Rezende NA, Blumberg HM, Metzger BS, Larsen NM, Ray SM, Mc Gowan JE Jr. Risk factors for methicillin resistance among patients with *Staphylococcus aureus* bacteremia at the time of hospital admission. Am J Med Sci 2002; 323:117–123

22. Lodise TP Jr, McKinnon PS, Rybak M. Prediction model to identify patients with *Staphylococcus aureus* bacteremia at risk of methicillin resistance. Infect Control Hosp Epidemiol 2003; 24:655–661.

23. Siberry GK, Tekle T, Carroll K, Dick J. Failure of clindamycin treatment of methicillin-resistant *Staphylococcus aureus* expressing inducible clindamycin resistance in vitro. Clin Infect Dis 2003; 37:1257–1260.

24. Schrenzel J, Harbarth S, Schockmel G, et al. Swiss Staphylococcal Study Group. A randomized clinical trial to compare fleroxacin-rifampicin with flucloxacillin or vancomycin for the treatment of staphylococcal infection. Clin Infect Dis 2004; 39:1285–1292.

25. Itani KMF. Infections in the surgical patient: an update on trends and treatments. Am J Surg 2003; 186(5A):1S–3S.

26. Weigelt JA, Itani KMF, Stevens D, Lau WK, Dryden M, Knirsch C. Linezolid vs vancomycin in the treatment of complicated skin and soft tissue infections. Antimicrob Agents Ch 2005; 49(6):1–7.

27. Weigelt J, Kaafarani HMA, Itani KMF, Swanson RN. Linezolid eradicates MRSA better than vancomycin from surgical-site infections. Am J Surg 2004; 188:760–766.

28. Itani KMF, Weigelt J, Li JZ, Duttagupta S. Linezolid reduces length of stay and intravenous therapy duration compared with vancomycin for complicated skin and soft tissue infections due to suspected methicillin resistant *Staphylococcus aureus*. Int J Antimicrob Agents 2005; 26(6):442–448.

29. Mc Kinnon PS, Sorensen S, Liu L, Itani KMF. The impact of linezolid on economic outcomes and determinants of cost in patients with documented or suspected MRSA complicated skin and soft-tissue infections. Annals of Pharmacotherapy 2006; 40(6):1017–1023.

30. Arbeit RD, Maki D, Tally FP, Campanaro E, Eisenstein BI; Daptomycin 98-01 and 99-01 Investigators. The safety and efficacy of daptomycin for the treatment of complicated skin and skin-structure infections. Clin Infect Dis 2004; 38:1673–1681.

31. Breedt J, Teras J, Gardovskis J, et al.; Tigecycline 305 cSSSI Study Group. Safety and efficacy of tigecycline in treatment of skin and skin structure infections: results of a double-blind phase 3 comparison study with vancomycin-aztreonam. Antimicrob Agents Chemother 2005; 49(11):4658–4666.

MRSA in the Diabetic Foot

6

Lee C. Rogers, Nicholas J. Bevilacqua, and
David G. Armstrong
The Center for Lower Extremity Ambulatory Research (CLEAR),
Dr. William M. Scholl College of Podiatric Medicine,
Rosalind Franklin University of Medicine and Science,
Chicago, Illinois, U.S.A.

DIABETIC FOOT: THE SCOPE OF THE PROBLEM

Diabetic foot problems remain a major burden on healthcare resources.
Diabetic foot ulcers (DFU) affect up to 25% of diabetics during their life-
time. Diabetic foot ulcers/infections are the most common reason for
hospitalization among diabetic patients in the United States (1). Hospital
length of stay is 59% longer for diabetic patients with ulcers when compared
to those without ulcers (2). Foot ulcers are the antecedent event in 84% of
diabetic lower extremity amputations (LEA) (3). More than half of the
approximately 120,000 nontraumatic amputations each year are performed
on people with diabetes, making diabetes the leading cause of nontraumatic
amputations (4). The Centers for Disease Control 1999 Surveillance
Summary for nontraumatic amputations revealed that LEAs increased by
24% between 1983 and 1996. There were 10.2 LEAs per 1000 diabetic
patients (5). Infection precedes 59% of diabetic amputations (3).

A person with diabetes and one LEA has a 50% chance of develop-
ing a limb-threatening condition on the contralateral limb within two years
(6). Diabetics with foot problems are at increased risk of mortality.
Jeffcoate et al. followed 449 diabetic patients with ulcers for 12 months.
Only 45% were alive, without amputation, and ulcer free at the endpoint.
A total of 11% of patients had undergone some form of amputation and

71

17% had died (7). Ramsey et al. (8) reviewed 8905 patients with diabetes, the cumulative three-year survival rate was 72% for patients with a foot ulcer versus 87% for those without ulcers. Lavery et al. (9) followed 1666 patients with diabetes for an average of 27 months. Ulcerations developed in 247 patients and infections in 151 patients, with an infection to ulcer ratio of 0.56.

The diagnosis of diabetic foot infection (DFI) is primarily based on the clinical examination. Diagnosis is made by the presence of purulence or two or more of the following signs/symptoms: erythema, induration, pain, tenderness, or warmth (10). Laboratory testing is of little use in the diagnosis of foot infections in diabetic patients. Leukocytosis is only present in 46% of diabetic patients with moderate to severe DFIs (11). Diabetics have blunted immune responses with abnormalities in granulocyte adherence, chemotaxis, and phagocytosis. Plasma glucose levels greater than 220 mg/dL in diabetics on day 1 after surgery is associated with a 30% postoperative infection rate (12).

O'Meara et al. (13) concluded that no evidence was available to describe the optimal methods of diagnosing a foot infection in a diabetic population. The Infectious Disease Society of America did publish guidelines for diagnosing DFI with a classification system for presence and extent of infection (Table 1) (14). Another commonly used, simple classification is non-limb-threatening or limb-threatening DFI (15). Non-limb-threatening infections have less than 2 cm of surrounding cellulitis, whereas limb-threatening infections have more extensive cellulitis. The University of Texas Diabetic Foot Ulcer Classification scheme is a useful tool to classify DFU based on depth, presence/absence of infection, and ischemia (16). Although not a direct classification of DFI per se, it is highly prognostic for amputation (17).

The diagnosis of osteomyelitis (OM) in DFIs is difficult and controversial. Grayson et al. (18) reported that palpating bone with a sterile blunt metal instrument inserted into a wound had a positive predictive value of 89% for OM; however, their study population had a high pretest probability of OM. This may have lead to the overrepresentation of OM in

TABLE 1 Classification of Diabetic Foot Infections

Clinical description	IDSA class	Caputo class
No signs or symptoms of infection	Uninfected	N/A
Surrounding cellulitis ≤2 cm, infection limited to skin and superficial soft-tissue, no systemic signs, or symptoms	Mild	Non-limb-threatening
Surrounding cellulitis >2 cm, systemically stable and may have lymphangitis, abscess, gangrene, or osteomyelitis	Moderate	Limb-threatening
Infection with signs or symptoms of systemic toxicity or in a patient who is medically unstable	Severe	

Abbreviation: IDSA, Infectious Disease Society of America.
Source: From Refs. 14, 15.

their study (19). El-Maghraby et al. (20) recently published a thorough review on the accuracy of a variety of imaging modalities that exist to diagnose OM. They reported that plain radiographs have a sensitivity and specificity of 43% to 75% and 75% to 83%, respectively. Scintigraphic methods were reviewed and Tech[99] triphasic bone scans had a sensitivity of 73% to 100%. Tech[99] scans are not very specific and can be "hot" (positive) with any number of bone pathologies such as fracture, postsurgical osteotomies, tumors, periosteal inflammation/bruising, or Charcot foot. Galium[67] citrate scans were more specific for infection with a specificity as high as 92%. White blood cell labeled bone scans (In[111] or HMPAO) had sensitivities and specificities in the range of 80% to 90%. Magnetic resonance imaging (MRI) had a sensitivity/specificity for OM as high as 100%/96%. MRI has difficulty when assessing for OM in the smaller bones in the foot.

Appropriate antibiotic therapy of a DFI usually requires culturing the wound and performing sensitivity testing on isolated pathogens (21,22). However, a wound culture is not to be used to diagnose wound infection, but rather to direct the therapy. Emphasis on a proper wound culture technique is paramount. Uninfected wounds should not be cultured. The accuracy of a wound culture depends on obtaining an appropriate specimen (21). There are several different techniques used for obtaining tissue samples from the wound including superficial swab cultures, needle aspiration, and wound biopsy. Superficial swab cultures are often used in the clinical setting, as some believe that they are cost-effective, less invasive, and adequately diagnostic (10). There is inconsistency in the literature whether a superficial swab culture reflects surface flora only or the causative pathogens (23–25). A proper wound culture should be obtained after debridement of all infected and necrotic tissue. This requires careful attention to sterile technique as well as selection of the optimal portion of the wound for sampling (22,26). Deep, initially unexposed, tissue removed with sterile instruments will generally yield the most accurate culture results (27). It is important to obtain both aerobic and anaerobic cultures of the wound. Once the cultures are sent, the patient should be started empirically on antibiotics.

The microbiology of DFIs generally depends on the severity of the infection. Non-limb-threatening infections are usually the result of gram-positive bacteria, predominately *S. aureus* and *Streptococcus* spp. (28). Limb-threatening infections tend to be polymicrobial with a mixture of gram-positive, gram-negative, aerobic, and anaerobic bacteria. An average of 2.8 to 5.8 bacteria are cultured from these infections (10,29,30).

MSRA IN DIABETIC FOOT INFECTIONS

Previous reports found up to 30% of skin isolates were methicillin-resistant *S. aureus* (MRSA) (31). Tentolouris et al. looked at MRSA prevalence in infected and uninfected DFUs. *S. aureus* was the most common pathogen and almost 50% were methicillin-resistant (32). Dang et al. (33) evaluated wound swab cultures in 63 outpatients with diabetes and foot ulcers, and found that gram-positive bacteria predominated in 84.2% (*S. aureus* in 79%). MRSA was cultured in 30.2%, which is an increase of almost double from their previous report only three years earlier (34). Similarly, in 911 patients with chronic ulcers, Roghmann (35) found that 30% were colonized with MRSA.

Risk factors for MRSA infections include recent previous hospitalization (36–38), nursing home residence (38,39), and prior antibiotic usage (39,40), but perhaps the single most important risk factor is a previous history of MRSA infection/colonization (39–41). Huang and Platt reported that the 18-month risk of reinfection with MRSA in 209 patients was 29%. Twenty-eight percent of those infections involved bacteremia and 56% involved pneumonia, soft-tissue, OM, or septic arthritis (41). Risk factors for MRSA infection in orthopedic and burn patient admissions were previous hospital stay within three months, the use of broad-spectrum antibiotics in the past two weeks, and previous infection/carriage of MRSA. Sixty-two percent of the patients with a previous history of MRSA developed reinfection (40).

Patients with diabetes have increased morbidity and mortality from MRSA infections. Diabetes is associated with persistent bacteremia in patients with MRSA (42). Patients whose wounds are colonized with MRSA have a risk ratio of 16 for developing MRSA bacteremia (35). MRSA bacteremia is associated with a 43% mortality rate compared with 20% for methicillin-sensitive *S. aureus* (MSSA) bacteremia (43). Tsao et al. infected diabetic and nondiabetic mice with MSSA and MRSA. Diabetic mice infected with MRSA died at an average of 10.6 (± 0.7) days, whereas nondiabetic mice infected with MRSA died at 19.1 (± 1.4) days. MSSA infections did not cause death in either group of mice. Diabetic mice infected with MRSA had significant increases in C-reactive protein, fibrinogen, fibronectin, and von Willebrand factor over nondiabetic mice. The authors concluded that MRSA infections in diabetic mice accelerated the inflammatory process, endothelial injury, and blood coagulation, ultimately leading to a quicker death (44). Additionally, there are case reports of MRSA causing necrotizing fasciitis in patients with diabetes (45,46).

Diabetic outcomes are worse in patients with MRSA infections, and hospital length of stay is longer for these patients (35). Grimble et al. (47) reviewed 30 patients undergoing major amputation. Seventeen of 30 amputated limbs had cultures positive for MRSA. Mortality was 43% in patients with MRSA-infected limbs compared with only 9% in nonMRSA infections. Primary healing was achieved in only four of 17 (24%) amputations with MRSA infections. Richards et al. (48) prospectively followed 25 patients with 33 primary amputations (14 above the knee and 19 below the knee). At time of surgery, 45% of the legs were colonized or infected with MRSA. Postoperative stump infection developed in 24% of patients, 71% of which were MRSA infections.

CLINICAL APPROACH TO TREATMENT OF DIABETIC FOOT INFECTIONS

Adequate débridement is perhaps the most important initial treatment of diabetic wound infections. Devitalized tissue in a wound can delay healing, predispose to infection, and interfere with adequate assessment (49–51). Debridement, by definition, is removing necrotic tissue, foreign material, and infecting bacteria from a wound (52). The goal is to excise the wound completely until only normal, soft, and well-vascularized tissue remains (52). Surgical debridement may be necessary for limb-threatening infections, whereas clinic debridement can be performed in non-limb-threatening infections. Debridement is performed using various instruments and techniques. A surgical blade is used to debride the borders of the wound, and excise the fibrotic and necrotic tissue within the wound base. Tissue nippers are used to remove any undermining, and a curette is used to remove the overlying proteinaceous coagulum at the base of the wound. The wound is debrided until only healthy, bleeding tissue is present. The role of debridement is to convert an infected, fibrotic wound to a healthy granular wound.

Over the past decades, there have been numerous biotechnological advances in wound healing modalities, including the development of acellular-matrix-based materials, cytokines, and bioengineered tissue replacements. All of these advanced technologies can only be considered when the wound is uninfected and well-vascularized with granular tissue. These modalities enhance granulation tissue, and ultimately ease the transition to wound closure by secondary intention, delayed primary closure, or skin grafting.

The use of negative pressure wound therapy (NPWT) with the WOUND V.A.C.® (KCI, San Antonio, Texas, U.S.A.) is, in large part, responsible for simplifying wound care, because it helps promote granulation tissue formation so that the wound size becomes manageable (52). NPWT applies localized negative pressure to help uniformly draw wounds closed. It has a cellular microdeformational effect, which helps remove interstitial fluid and infectious material. The V.A.C. provides a closed, moist wound healing environment and helps promote flap and graft survival (53). A multicenter, randomized, controlled trial compared NPWT to standard moist wound care after partial diabetic foot amputation. The rate of wound healing and granulation tissue formation was faster in the NPWT group compared to the controls. Both groups had similar frequency and severity of adverse events (54).

Cell-based technologies help deliver exogenous growth factors to the wound bed. Two Food and Drug Administration (FDA)-approved products are APLIGRAF® and DERMAGRAFT®. Extracellular matrix scaffolds help organize the healing process and provide a scaffolding for the host cells to grow. These include GRAFTJACKET® Matrix, INTEGRA® BMD, OASIS® (noncrosslinked xenograft), and GAMMAGRAFT™ (irradiated cadaveric skin). Isolated recombinant growth factors, like platelet-derived growth factor in REGRANEX® can be used to promote granulation tissue.

Offloading of the involved foot is a key component of treating a DFU. A vascularized, uninfected, granular wound will not heal unless the mechanical forces are reduced or eliminated. There are many offloading modalities including bed rest, wheel chair, crutches, total contact casts (TCCs), removable cast walkers (RCWs), instant total contact cast (iTCC), half shoes, custom splints, and therapeutic shoes. Crutches are not advocated, since diabetics with peripheral diseases have other central diseases and crutch walking increases the energy of ambulation. These patients may not have adequate cardiac reserves for ambulating with crutches. In addition, diabetics with peripheral neuropathy have sensory ataxia and may risk falling while attempting to use crutches. A Roll-A-Bout® (Roll-A-Bout Corp., Federica, Maryland, U.S.A.) is a "rolling crutch," which allows offloading of the foot while the healthy extremity propels the device and may be useful in these patients. Wheelchairs are effective pressure reduction devices; however, most patients' homes are not designed to accommodate the bulkiness of the wheelchairs and this can lead to high levels of noncompliant activity (55). The TCC is effective because it permits walking while offloading by uniformly distributing pressures over the entire plantar surface of the foot (56,57). However, applying the TCC is technically demanding and requires training and experience. The biggest drawback to TCC is that improper cast application can cause skin irritation and frank ulceration. RCWs offer several potential advantages over the traditional TCC. Data from gait lab studies suggest that the amount of pressure reduction for certain RCWs is equivalent to TCCs (58). They are, as their name implies, removable, which is their greatest drawback. Patients simply do not use them during all ambulatory activities. One study found that patients only wore their removable offloading device for less than 30% of their total daily activity (59). Armstrong et al. suggested a potential alternative, a RCW made less removable. This simple concept, termed an "iTCC" (60), involves simply wrapping the RCW with either a layer of cohesive bandage or plaster/fiberglass, thereby making it more difficult for patients to remove. The iTCC may have the benefit of adequate offloading (on par with the TCC) as well as "forced adherence" to the prescribed course of pressure reduction.

MODIFICATION OF ANTIMICROBIAL TREATMENT IN THE ERA OF MRSA

Initial empiric therapy of non-limb-threatening infections, being primarily gram-positive, consists of oral outpatient therapy utilizing medications such as cephalexin, amoxicillin/clavulanate, or clindamycin. More severe limb-threatening infections should be treated with inpatient intra-veneous therapies including piperacillin/tazobactam (61), ertapenem (62), imipenem, or a fluorquinolone. Upon review of the culture and sen-sitivity, de-escalation and targeted antibiotic therapy should be initiated. The question, which remains unanswered, is at what point should physicians begin including antibiotics active against MRSA in their empiric therapy? As was presented in this chapter, the prevalence of MRSA infections/colonization in diabetic feet is increasing drastically. If empiric coverage is to be considered, it should be implemented for limb-threatening infections as well as non-limb-threatening infections, since they are predominately *S. aureus* isolates.

Vancomycin, daptomycin, linezolid, tigecycline, and quinupristin-dalfopristin have all been studied for skin and soft-tissue infections. Vancomycin has been the historical drug of choice for MRSA DFIs. Its use has been questioned with the emerging vancomycin-resistant *S. aureus* (VRSA) and vancomycin-resistant *Enterococcus* (VRE). Chronic ulcers and vancomycin use place one at risk for developing VRSA (63). Although vancomycin is commonly used for diabetic foot OM with MRSA, one study evaluating vancomycin for vertebral OM reported that vancomycin alone was not sufficient for resolution (64).

Daptomycin is a lipopeptide antibiotic active against VRE, MRSA, glycopeptide-intermediate susceptible *S. aureus*, and coagulase-negative staphylococci (65). It is FDA approved for use in complicated skin and skin-structure infections (cSSSI) (31). Daptomycin has been studied in infected DFU and found to be equivalent to vancomycin or a semisynthetic penicillin (66). Some staphylococcal resistance has recently been reported to daptomycin (67). An in vitro OM model measuring the leeching of antibiotic for vancomycin and daptomycin revealed that both drugs were similar in concentration released (68).

Quinupristin/dalfopristin is a parenteral streptogramin antimicrobial agent with activity against a broad range of gram-positive bacteria including MRSA, VRE, *Streptococci*, *Clostridium perfringens*, and *Peptostreptococcus* spp. (69). It is approved for severe or life-threatening infections associated with VRE. Quinupristin/dalfopristin has not been evaluated for use in DFIs.

Tigecycline is a glycylcycline antibiotic related to the tetracycline group of drugs. It is broad-spectrum with activity against MRSA, VRE, and multiple gram-negative bacteria, excluding *Pseudomonas* spp. (70). It has been shown to be equivalent to vancomycin plus aztreonam in cSSSI (71). In experimental OM with a rabbit model, tigeclycline plus rifampin showed 100% clearance of OM in four weeks, compared with vancomycin plus rifampin at 90%, and only 26% in the untreated controls (72).

Linezolid, an oxazolidinone, is broadly active against gram-positive bacteria including MRSA and VRE, and is FDA-approved for a complicated skin and soft-tissue infection (cSSTI) (73). Linezolid is the only antibiotic with activity against MRSA to have an FDA indication for DFIs. Unlike the other anti-MRSA drugs, linezolid is available in parenteral and oral forms, with the oral formation having 100% bioavailability (74). Stevens et al. (75) randomized 460 patients with known or suspected MRSA cSSTI to linezolid or vancomycin. There was no statistical difference between the clinical cure rates. Weigelt et al. (76) found superior outcomes with linezolid at a test of cure visit for cSSTI, when compared with vancomycin in 285 patients. Another study (77), randomizing 1200 patients with cSSSI suspected or known to be MRSA, found linezolid greatly reduced the length of hospital stay and the duration of parenteral antibiotics. McKinnon et al. (78) evaluated the economic outcomes of linezolid versus vancomycin, and also found that length of stay and costs were reduced with linezolid. Specifically evaluating lower extremity cSSTI caused by MRSA, Sharp et al. found a greater cure rate and an average of three-day shorter length of stay for linezolid versus vancomycin. Vancomycin was associated with more treatment failures and major amputations (79). In OM, linezolid plus surgical resection and reconstruction was associated with a 90% success rate in 40 patients (80). Rayner et al. (81) found that linezolid was effective in the treatment of OM with an 82% cure rate, however, only 22 of 89 patients were available for follow-up.

CONCLUSIONS

The burden of MRSA in DFIs is increasing, causing more treatment failures, increased length of hospital stays, increased healthcare costs, and more amputations. MRSA DFIs are associated with greater morbidity and mortality. There is a paucity of literature evaluating the treatment of MRSA infections specifically in DFIs. Linezolid seems to have the greatest amount of evidence and the most patients studied. Being available in intravenous and oral formulations is another advantage to using linezolid, allowing quicker discharge of hospital patients. No sufficient evidence exists regarding the use of any anti-MRSA drug in the setting of OM, which forces physicians to choose one based on anecdote or safety/adverse effect profile. Caution must be taken as bacterial resistance to these new drugs will develop, especially when being used in the environment of a chronic skin ulcer. Rapid identification of DFI, de-escalating culture-directed antimicrobial therapy, and addressing the concomitant conditions that delay wound healing can help to prevent LEA in this high-risk population.

REFERENCES

1. Singh N, Armstrong DG, Lipsky BA. Preventing foot ulcers in patients with diabetes. JAMA 2005; 293(2):217–228.

2. Reiber GE, Boyko EJ, Smith DG. Lower extremity foot ulcers and amputations in diabetes. In: Harris MI, Cowie C, Stern MP, eds. Diabetes in America. 2nd ed. Washington, DC: United Government Printing Office (NIH Publ. 95–1468), 1995.

3. Pecoraro RE, Reiber GE, Burgess EM. Pathways to diabetic limb amputation: basis for prevention. Diabetes Care 1990; 13:513–521.

4. Armstrong DG, Lavery LA. Diabetic foot ulcers: prevention, diagnosis and classification. Am Fam Phys 1998; 57:1325–1340.

5. Control CfD. Surveillance Summary; Non-traumatic Amputations. www.cdc.gov/diabetes/statistics/survl99/chap1/amputations.htm. Accessed September 6, 2006.

6. Goldner MG. The fate of the second leg in the diabetic amputee. Diabetes 1960; 9:100–103.

7. Jeffcoate WJ, Chipchase SY, Ince P, Game FL. Assessing the outcome of the management of diabetic foot ulcers using ulcer-related and person-related measures. Diabetes Care 2006; 29(8):1784–1787.

8. Ramsey SD, Newton K, Blough D, et al. Incidence, outcomes, and cost of foot ulcers in patients with diabetes. Diabetes Care 1999; 22(3):382–387.

9. Lavery LA, Armstrong DG, Wunderlich RP, Mohler MJ, Wendel CS, Lipsky BA. Risk factors for foot infections in individuals with diabetes. Diabetes Care 2006; 29(6):1288–1293.

10. Karchmer AW. Microbiology and treatment of diabetic foot infections. In: Veves A, Giurini JM, LoGerfo FW, eds. The Diabetic Foot. 2nd ed. Totowa, New Jersey: Humana Press, 2006:255–268.

11. Armstrong DG, Lavery LA, Sariaya M, Ashry H. Leukocytosis is a poor indicator of acute osteomyelitis of the foot in diabetes mellitus. J Foot Ankle Surg 1996; 35(4):280–283.

12. McMahon MM, Bistrian BR. Host defenses and susceptibility to infection in patients with diabetes mellitus. Infect Dis Clin North Am 1995; 9(1):1–9.

13. O'Meara S, Nelson EA, Golder S, Dalton JE, Craig D, Iglesias C. Systematic review of methods to diagnose infection in foot ulcers in diabetes. Diabet Med 2006; 23(4):341–347.

14. Lipsky BA, Berendt AR, Deery HG, et al. Diagnosis and treatment of diabetic foot infections. Clin Infect Dis 2004; 39(7):885–910.

15. Caputo GM, Cavanagh PR, Ulbrecht JS, Gibbons GW, Karchmer AW. Assessment and management of foot disease in patients with diabetes. N Engl J Med 1994; 331(13):854–860.

16. Armstrong DG, Lavery LA, Harkless LB. Validation of a diabetic wound classification system. The contribution of depth, infection, and ischemia to risk of amputation [see comments]. Diabetes Care 1998; 21(5):855–859.
17. Oyibo SO, Jude EB, Tarawneh I, et al. A comparison of two diabetic foot ulcer classification systems. Diabetes 2000; 49(suppl 1):A33.
18. Grayson ML, Balaugh K, Levin E, Karchmer AW. Probing to bone in infected pedal ulcers. A clinical sign of underlying osteomyelitis in diabetic patients. J Am Med Assoc 1995; 273(9):721–723.
19. Shone A, Burnside J, Chipchase S, Game F, Jeffcoate W. Probing the validity of the probe-to-bone test in the diagnosis of osteomyelitis of the foot in diabetes. Diabetes Care 2006; 29(4):945.
20. El-Maghraby TA, Moustafa HM, Pauwels EK. Nuclear medicine methods for evaluation of skeletal infection among other diagnostic modalities. Q J Nucl Med Mol Imaging 2006; 50(3):167–192.
21. Lipsky BA. A current approach to diabetic foot infections. Curr Infect Dis Rep 1999; 1(3):253–260.
22. Neil JA, Munro CL. A comparison of two culturing methods for chronic wounds. Ostomy Wound Manage 1997; 43(3):20–22, 24, 26 passim.
23. Wheat LJ, Allen SD, Henry M, et al. Diabetic foot infections. Bacteriologic analysis. Arch Intern Med 1986; 146(10):1935–1940.
24. Slater RA, Lazarovitch T, Boldur I, et al. Swab cultures accurately identify bacterial pathogens in diabetic foot wounds not involving bone. Diabet Med 2004; 21(7):705–709.
25. Pellizzer G, Strazzabosco M, Presi S, et al. Deep tissue biopsy vs. superficial swab culture monitoring in the microbiological assessment of limb-threatening diabetic foot infection. Diabet Med 2001; 18(10):822–827.
26. Calhoun JH, Overgaard KA, Stevens CM, Dowling JP, Mader JT. Diabetic foot ulcers and infections: current concepts. Adv Skin Wound Care 2002; 15(1):31–42; quiz 44–35.
27. Williams DT, Hilton JR, Harding KG. Diagnosing foot infection in diabetes. Clin Infect Dis 2004; 39(suppl 2):S83–S86.
28. Lipsky BA. Medical treatment of diabetic foot infections. Clin Infect Dis 2004; 39(suppl 2):S104–S114.
29. Grayson ML, Gibbons GW, Habershaw GM, et al. Use of ampicillin/sulbactam versus imipenem/cilastatin in the treatment of limb-threatening foot infections in diabetic patients. Clin Infect Dis 1994; 18(5):683–693.
30. Scher KS, Steele FJ. The septic foot in patients with diabetes. Surgery 1988; 104:661–666.

31. LaPlante KL, Rybak MJ. Daptomycin—a novel antibiotic against gram-positive pathogens. Expert Opin Pharmacother 2004; 5(11):2321–2331.

32. Tentolouris N, Petrikkos G, Vallianou N, et al. Prevalence of methicillin-resistant *Staphylococcus aureus* in infected and uninfected diabetic foot ulcers. Clin Microbiol Infect 2006; 12(2):186–189.

33. Dang CN, Prasad YD, Boulton AJ, Jude EB. Methicillin-resistant *Staphylococcus aureus* in the diabetic foot clinic: a worsening problem. Diabet Med 2003; 20(2):159–161.

34. Tentolouris N, Jude EB, Smirnof I, Knowles EA, Boulton AJ. Methicillin-resistant *Staphylococcus aureus*: an increasing problem in a diabetic foot clinic. Diabet Med 1999; 16(9):767–771.

35. Roghmann MC, Siddiqui A, Plaisance K, Standiford H. MRSA colonization and the risk of MRSA bacteraemia in hospitalized patients with chronic ulcers. J Hosp Infect 2001; 47(2):98–103.

36. Warshawsky B, Hussain Z, Gregson DB, et al. Hospital- and community-based surveillance of methicillin-resistant *Staphylococcus aureus*: previous hospitalization is the major risk factor. Infect Control Hosp Epidemiol 2000; 21(11):724–727.

37. Jernigan JA, Pullen AL, Flowers L, Bell M, Jarvis WR. Prevalence of and risk factors for colonization with methicillin-resistant *Staphylococcus aureus* at the time of hospital admission. Infect Control Hosp Epidemiol 2003; 24(6):409–414.

38. Furuno JP, Harris AD, Wright MO, et al. Prediction rules to identify patients with methicillin-resistant *Staphylococcus aureus* and vancomycin-resistant enterococci upon hospital admission. Am J Infect Control 2004; 32(8): 436–440.

39. Troillet N, Carmeli Y, Samore MH, et al. Carriage of methicillin-resistant *Staphylococcus aureus* at hospital admission. Infect Control Hosp Epidemiol 1998; 19(3):181–185.

40. Vidhani S, Mathur MD, Mehndiratta PL, Rizvi M. Methicillin resistant *Staphylococcus aureus* (MRSA): the associated risk factors. Indian J Pathol Microbiol 2003; 46(4):676–679.

41. Huang SS, Platt R. Risk of methicillin-resistant *Staphylococcus aureus* infection after previous infection or colonization. Clin Infect Dis 2003; 36(3):281–285.

42. Khatib R, Johnson LB, Fakih MG, et al. Persistence in *Staphylococcus aureus* bacteremia: incidence, characteristics of patients and outcome. Scand J Infect Dis 2006; 38(1):7–14.

43. Talon D, Woronoff-Lemsi MC, Limat S, et al. The impact of resistance to methicillin in *Staphylococcus aureus* bacteremia on mortality. Eur J Intern Med 2002; 13(1):31–36.

44. Tsao SM, Hsu CC, Yin MC. Meticillin-resistant *Staphylococcus aureus* infection in diabetic mice enhanced inflammation and coagulation. J Med Microbiol 2006; 55(pt 4):379–385.

45. Miller LG, Perdreau-Remington F, Rieg G, et al. Necrotizing fasciitis caused by community-associated methicillin-resistant *Staphylococcus aureus* in Los Angeles. N Engl J Med 2005; 352(14):1445–1453.

46. Wong CH, Tan SH, Kurup A, Tan AB. Recurrent necrotizing fasciitis caused by methicillin-resistant *Staphylococcus aureus*. Eur J Clin Microbiol Infect Dis 2004; 23(12):909–911.

47. Grimble SA, Magee TR, Galland RB. Methicillin resistant *Staphylococcus aureus* in patients undergoing major amputation. Eur J Vasc Endovasc Surg 2001; 22(3):215–218.

48. Richards T, Pittathankel AA, Pursell R, Magee TR, Galland RB. MRSA in lower limb amputation and the role of antibiotic prophylaxis. J Cardiovasc Surg (Torino) 2005; 46(1):37–41.

49. Boulton AJ, Meneses P, Ennis WJ. Diabetic foot ulcers: a framework for prevention and care. Wound Repair Regen 1999; 7(1):7–16.

50. Rauwerda JA. Foot debridement: anatomic knowledge is mandatory. Diabetes Metab Res Rev 2000; 16(suppl 1):S23–S26.

51. Sibbald RG, Williamson D, Orsted HL, et al. Preparing the wound bed–debridement, bacterial balance, and moisture balance. Ostomy Wound Manage 2000; 46(11):14–22, 24–18, 30–15; quiz 36–17.

52. Attinger CE, Bulan EJ. Debridement. The key initial first step in wound healing. Foot Ankle Clin 2001; 6(4):627–660.

53. Saxena V, Hwang CW, Huang S, Eichbaum Q, Ingber D, Orgill DP. Vacuum-assisted closure: microdeformations of wounds and cell proliferation. Plast Reconstr Surg 2004; 114(5):1086–1096; discussion 1097–1088.

54. Armstrong DG, Lavery LA. Negative pressure wound therapy after partial diabetic foot amputation: a multicentre, randomised controlled trial. Lancet 2005; 366(9498):1704–1710.

55. Wu SC, Crews RT, Armstrong DG. The pivotal role of offloading in the management of neuropathic foot ulceration. Curr Diab Rep 2005; 5(6):423–429.

56. Armstrong DG, Lavery LA, Bushman TR. Peak foot pressures influence healing time of diabetic ulcers treated with total contact casting. J Rehabil Res Dev 1998; 35:1–5.

57. Sinacore DR, Mueller MJ, Diamond JE. Diabetic plantar ulcers treated by total contact casting. Phys Ther 1987; 67:1543–1547.

58. Lavery LA, Vela SA, Lavery DC, Quebedeaux TL. Reducing dynamic foot pressures in high-risk diabetic subjects with foot ulcerations. A comparison of treatments. Diabetes Care 1996; 19(8):818–821.

59. Armstrong DG, Lavery LA, Kimbriel HR, Nixon BP, Boulton AJ. Activity patterns of patients with diabetic foot ulceration: Patients with active ulceration may not adhere to a standard pressure off-loading regimen. Diabetes Care 2003; 26(9):2595–2597.

60. Armstrong DG, Short B, Nixon BP, Boulton AJM. Technique for fabrication of an "instant" total contact cast for treatment of neuropathic diabetic foot ulcers. J Amer Podiatr Med Assn 2002; 92:405–408.

61. Harkless L, Boghossian J, Pollak R, et al. An open-label, randomized study comparing efficacy and safety of intravenous piperacillin/tazobactam and ampicillin/sulbactam for infected diabetic foot ulcers. Surg Infect (Larchmt) 2005; 6(1):27–40.

62. Lipsky BA, Armstrong DG, Citron DM, Tice AD, Morgenstern DE, Abramson MA. Ertapenem versus piperacillin/tazobactam for diabetic foot infections (SIDESTEP): prospective, randomised, controlled, double-blinded, multi-centre trial. Lancet 2005; 366(9498):1695–1703.

63. Appelbaum PC. The emergence of vancomycin-intermediate and vancomycin-resistant *Staphylococcus aureus*. Clin Microbiol Infect 2006; 12(suppl 1):16–23.

64. Gelfand MS, Cleveland KO. Vancomycin therapy and the progression of methicillin-resistant *Staphylococcus aureus* vertebral osteomyelitis. South Med J 2004; 97(6):593–597.

65. Tally FP, Zeckel M, Wasilewski MM, et al. Daptomycin: a novel agent for Gram-positive infections. Expert Opin Investig Drugs 1999; 8(8): 1223–1238.

66. Lipsky BA, Stoutenburgh U. Daptomycin for treating infected diabetic foot ulcers: evidence from a randomized, controlled trial comparing daptomycin with vancomycin or semi-synthetic penicillins for compli-cated skin and skin-structure infections. J Antimicrob Chemother 2005; 55(2):240–245.

67. Jevitt LA, Thorne GM, Traczewski MM, et al. Multicenter evaluation of the Etest and disk diffusion methods for differentiating daptomycin-susceptible from non-daptomycin-susceptible *Staphylococcus aureus* isolates. J Clin Microbiol 2006; 44(9):3098–3104.

68. Rouse MS, Piper KE, Jacobson M, Jacofsky DJ, Steckelberg JM, Patel R. Daptomycin treatment of *Staphylococcus aureus* experimental chronic osteomyelitis. J Antimicrob Chemother 2006; 57(2):301–305.

69. Lamb HM, Figgitt DP, Faulds D. Quinupristin/dalfopristin: a review of its use in the management of serious gram-positive infections. Drugs 1999; 58(6):1061–1097.
70. Livermore DM. Tigecycline: what is it, and where should it be used? J Antimicrob Chemother 2005; 56(4):611–614.
71. Ellis-Grosse EJ, Babinchak T, Dartois N, Rose G, Loh E. The efficacy and safety of tigecycline in the treatment of skin and skin-structure infections: results of 2 double-blind phase 3 comparison studies with vancomycin-aztreonam. Clin Infect Dis 2005; 41(suppl 5):S341–S353.
72. Yin LY, Lazzarini L, Li F, Stevens CM, Calhoun JH. Comparative evaluation of tigecycline and vancomycin, with and without rifampicin, in the treatment of methicillin-resistant *Staphylococcus aureus* experimental osteomyelitis in a rabbit model. J Antimicrob Chemother 2005; 55(6):995–1002.
73. Peppard WJ, Weigelt JA. Role of linezolid in the treatment of complicated skin and soft tissue infections. Expert Rev Anti Infect Ther 2006; 4(3):357–366.
74. Plosker GL, Figgitt DP. Linezolid: a pharmacoeconomic review of its use in serious gram-positive infections. Pharmacoeconomics 2005; 23(9):945–964.
75. Stevens DL, Herr D, Lampiris H, Hunt JL, Batts DH, Hafkin B. Linezolid versus vancomycin for the treatment of methicillin-resistant *Staphylococcus aureus* infections. Clin Infect Dis 2002; 34(11):1481–1490.
76. Weigelt J, Itani K, Stevens D, Lau W, Dryden M, Knirsch C. Linezolid versus vancomycin in treatment of complicated skin and soft tissue infections. Antimicrob Agents Chemother 2005; 49(6):2260–2266.
77. Itani KM, Weigelt J, Li JZ, Duttagupta S. Linezolid reduces length of stay and duration of intravenous treatment compared with vancomycin for complicated skin and soft tissue infections due to suspected or proven methicillin-resistant *Staphylococcus aureus* (MRSA). Int J Antimicrob Agents 2005; 26(6):442–448.
78. McKinnon PS, Sorensen SV, Liu LZ, Itani KM. Impact of linezolid on economic outcomes and determinants of cost in a clinical trial evaluating patients with MRSA complicated skin and soft-tissue infections. Ann Pharmacother 2006; 40(6):1017–1023.
79. Sharpe JN, Shively EH, Polk HC Jr. Clinical and economic outcomes of oral linezolid versus intravenous vancomycin in the treatment of MRSA-complicated, lower-extremity skin and soft-tissue infections caused by methicillin-resistant *Staphylococcus aureus*. Am J Surg 2005; 189(4):425–428.
80. Broder KW, Moise PA, Schultz RO, Forrest A, Schentag JJ. Clinical experience with linezolid in conjunction with wound coverage techniques for skin

and soft-tissue infections and postoperative osteomyelitis. Ann Plast Surg 2004; 52(4):385–390.

81. Rayner CR, Baddour LM, Birmingham MC, Norden C, Meagher AK, Schentag JJ. Linezolid in the treatment of osteomyelitis: results of compassionate use experience. Infection 2004; 32(1):8–14.

MRSA Pneumonia

7

Anna P. Lam and Richard G. Wunderink
Division of Pulmonary and Critical Care Medicine,
Feinberg School of Medicine, Northwestern University,
Chicago, Illinois, U.S.A.

INTRODUCTION

Infections due to multi-drug resistant (MDR) organisms are a burgeoning problem in the treatment of increasingly complex medical patients. In particular, respiratory infections caused by methicillin-resistant *Staphylococcus aureus* (MRSA) are especially challenging. Whether acquired from the community or nosocomially, these highly adaptable bacteria possess distinctive genes for antibiotic resistance and toxins that present significant obstacles to effective care.

Pneumonia due to MRSA differs from infections with other MDR pathogens and pose unique challenges to successful treatment and prevention.

EPIDEMIOLOGY

Community-Acquired MRSA Pneumonia

Since the first description in a series of intravenous drug users at Henry Ford hospital in Detroit (1), reports of methicillin resistance in *S. aureus* isolates outside of healthcare facilities have been on the rise. Unlike nosocomial MRSA, community-acquired MRSA (CA-MRSA) is typically not MDR. However, this strain possesses leukocidin, a toxin first described by Panton and Valentine in 1932 (2). Panton–Valentine leukocidin (PVL) is rare, seen in less than 2% of all strains (3), but more likely to be found in community- than in hospital-acquired strains (4,5). In addition to other toxin genes, these PVL-positive isolates also carry the type IV SCC*mec* element characteristic of CA-MRSA, indicating that these isolates did not emerge from healthcare-associated pathogens (6,7). The genetic background of CA-MRSA isolates from various continents differ, suggesting simultaneous co-evolution rather than dissemination of a single clone (7).

Interest in PVL has been stimulated by the emergence of CA-MRSA strains carrying this toxin in necrotizing community-acquired pneumonias (CAPs) and skin infections (4,8,9). The CA-MRSA infections are found in younger patients and are more likely to involve skin and soft tissue than respiratory tract, compared to healthcare-associated MRSA (HA-MRSA) infections (5). However, CAP due to MRSA possessing PVL is increasingly reported, often associated with an antecedent influenza-like illness. Despite patients being young and otherwise healthy, these infections are associated with a mortality of up to 37% (6,8,10). Thus, early recognition and appropriate antibiotic therapy are essential for treatment of CA-MRSA pneumonia.

Healthcare-Acquired MRSA Pneumonia

S. aureus, both methicillin-sensitive (MSSA) and -resistant strains, is the most frequently isolated pathogen in the intensive care unit (ICU) (11). Patients with *S. aureus* infections had three times the length of stay and total charges and five times the risk of inpatient death as patients without *S. aureus* infections (12).

Ventilator-associated pneumonia (VAP) is not an uncommon complication for the ICU patient, with incidence rates from 1 to >20 cases per 1000 ventilator days (13). After five ICU days, VAP is more likely to be caused by MDR pathogens, including MRSA, which are associated with increased mortality rates (11,13–17). The incidence of MRSA as a cause of VAP is 12% to 15% overall, but increases to approximately 30% in patients with prolonged mechanical ventilation and prior antibiotic therapy (18). The incidence does vary from country to country, hospital to hospital (19,20), and even from ICU to ICU (21). Given the frequency of

MRSA as a cause of VAP, the initial treatment for VAP in most ICUs should include empiric vancomycin or linezolid (18,22,23).

Attributable mortality of nosocomial pneumonia in intubated and ventilated patients may be 27% with a risk ratio for death of 2.0 (15), although this is driven principally by mortality from non-fermenting gram-negative bacilli. The attributable mortality for MRSA may be closer to 15% to 20% (24–26). Mortality and attributable costs are consistently higher with MRSA VAP compared to MSSA (27–30).

The MRSA pneumonia, whether community-acquired or nosocomial, is a significant healthcare burden, requiring effective prevention and treatment strategies in order to decrease the associated mortality and morbidity. Despite limited therapeutic options, lively debate and controversy in this field abounds. Management has focused on risk factors, antibiotic therapy, and preventative measures.

RISK FACTORS FOR DEVELOPMENT OF MRSA PNEUMONIA

Nasal Carriage of *Staphylococcus aureus*

S. aureus is a human commensal organism that commonly colonizes the anterior nares. Up to 80% of the population are constant or intermittent carriers (31), including healthcare workers as well as patients. The bacteria can be carried in the nares for more than one year, with a half-life of colonization of MRSA around 40 months (32). Nasal carriage, rather than skin colonization, seems to be an important risk factor for invasive disease (31,33,34). This high frequency of colonization of both patients and their caregivers is unique from other MDR pathogens. In addition, nasal colonization requires prevention strategies different from gastrointestinal colonization or environmental contamination.

Prior Antibiotic Therapy

The major predisposing factor for CA-MRSA and HA-MRSA is prior antibiotic therapy (9,19,35). Antibiotic therapy is not a risk factor for MSSA infection. Early-onset MSSA VAP was found in only 14.6% of patients who did not receive prior antibiotics; none of these patients developed MRSA VAP (18). Even in those patients with prolonged (≥ 7 days) mechanical ventilation, the rate of MSSA VAP was 21.9% while MRSA VAP was only 3.1% if patients had not received any prior antibiotics. In contrast, 4.6% and 19.7% of patients developed MSSA VAP and MRSA VAP, respectively, when the patient had antibiotic exposure in the previous 15 days (18). Data from 17 U.S. hospitals showed a significant association between total inpatient fluoroquinolone use and percentage of MRSA isolated (36). Similar associations have been seen with macrolide and third-generation cephalosporin use (37).

Nursing home patients are more likely to have MRSA VAP. One of the major risk factors is prior antibiotic therapy, selecting for MDR pathogens in general (38). The increased percentage of MRSA in nursing homes correlates with increased quinolone but decreased trimethoprim-sulfamethoxazole use (39). Nasal carriage rates were also associated with prior antibiotic use in elderly residents of a nursing home (40).

Prolonged Mechanical Ventilation
The length of mechanical ventilation is a risk factor for development of MRSA VAP. During a five-year outbreak of MRSA, MRSA VAP only occurred after ≥ 3 ventilator days (41). While MRSA may cause early-onset VAP, the incidence of MRSA in late-onset (≥ 6 days) pneumonia is increased (14,27). Patients ventilated for more than 6 days have a two-fold relative risk for developing MRSA VAP (27).

Poor Infection Control
The emergence of antibiotic-resistant pathogens, including MRSA, is linked to breaches in infection control measures, such as noncompliance with hand-washing and isolation recommendations (11,42). Poor hygiene and infection control in military recruits and inmates resulted in MRSA outbreaks (43,44). More than two ICU patients having nasal MRSA colonization at the same time were associated with increased MRSA infections (45). Aggressive screening, contact precautions, and

use of alcoholic hand rub solutions in ICUs with a high prevalence of MRSA at admission reduced the spread to exposed patients (46).

Head Trauma/Coma

Patients with head injury and critically ill comatose patients are at increased risk for developing VAP (47,48). This event seems to occur before seven days in the course of mechanical ventilation (47,49,50). The most frequently isolated organism is *S. aureus* (48–50). Colonization of the nares, pharynx, and trachea with *S. aureus* was further associated with early-onset VAP in patients with head injuries (51–53).

Prior Viral Infection

The incidence of *S. aureus* CAP is increased during influenza epidemics. The new PVL-containing strains of CA-MRSA are associated with a preceding viral illness when presenting as pneumonia (6,8,10). Experimental rhinovirus infection also increases the shedding of *S. aureus* (54).

TREATMENT OPTIONS

Antimicrobial agents active against MRSA are limited. In the glycopeptide family, vancomycin is the best known in the United States. Teicoplanin is similar to vancomycin, but unavailable in the United States. These two glycopeptides have never undergone a randomized controlled trial to demonstrate their efficacy in MRSA pneumonia, yet they are the de facto standards since, until recently, no other viable alternatives existed.

Vancomycin/Teicoplanin

The efficacy of glycopeptide treatment for lower respiratory tract infections (LRTIs) remains controversial. Vancomycin intrinsically is less effective against Staphylococci than β-lactam antibiotics (55–57). Infection-associated mortality among patients with MSSA pneumonia was significantly higher for those treated with vancomycin than cloxacillin (47% vs. 0%, respectively) (28). Among patients with *S. aureus* LRTI, vancomycin clinical success was only 54%, even though 58% had MRSA, while all antibacterials other than vancomycin had a 71% clinical success rate, including a 100% clinical success rate in patients with MSSA pneumonia treated with oxacillin (58).

The clinical cure rates specifically for vancomycin treatment of MRSA hospital-acquired pneumonia (HAP) are shown in Figure 1 (35,59–61). No study has documented a clinical success rate greater than 65%, and significantly lower rates are found when only VAP is included. Inappropriate initial empiric therapy does not appear to be the reason for failure, since no difference in mortality was found even if vancomycin therapy was delayed up to 48 hours from the initial diagnosis (35).

Vancomycin is ineffective at clearing bacteria from the lower respiratory tract. Repeat quantitative cultures demonstrated that only 15% of patients with MRSA VAP treated with vancomycin had decreased

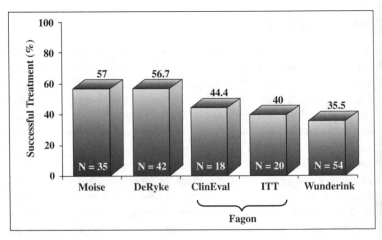

FIGURE 1 Clinical success of vancomycin treatment of MRSA ventilator-associated pneumonia.

colony counts below diagnostic thresholds (62). This finding contrasts with 85% sterile repeat cultures when VAP was due to other microorganisms. Failure to clear the bacteria within the first several days of treatment, not surprisingly, was associated with increased 28-day mortality (62).

One potential explanation for the poor clinical outcomes with vancomycin treatment of *S. aureus* pneumonia is the degree of penetration into lung tissue. Homogenized lung tissue from patients undergoing lung resection had low vancomycin levels compared to serum (lung to serum ratio 0.21) (63). By 3 hours postinfusion, a substantial portion of patients had lung vancomycin levels below the minimal inhibitory concentration (MIC), and at 12 hours postinfusion, almost half had no detectable level. In intubated patients with suspected pneumonia, the bronchoalveolar lavage (BAL) vancomycin concentration was only 25% of serum (64). More than half of MRSA VAP patients given vancomycin, 30 mg/kg, intravenously every 6 hours, had BAL vancomycin levels that were undetectable after four doses; in the remaining patients, mean BAL vancomycin concentration was 2.0 µg/mL with corresponding serum levels of 22.2 µg/mL and trough levels above 20 µg/mL (65).

One response to limited lung levels of vancomycin is to use more than two grams a day, which is the usual dose given. Higher doses of vancomycin, as measured by the area under the concentration curve (AUC), appeared to correlate with outcome (66). However, clinical success is also dependent on the MIC of the isolate. If the vancomycin MIC is 1 to 2 µg/mL, the success rate is less than 10% (67). An alternative is continuous infusion of vancomycin, which shows some promise (68). A multivariate analysis of outcomes from MRSA VAP suggests some benefit from a continuous infusion dosing strategy (26). Higher dosing or continuous infusion is more likely to be associated with renal toxicity. No prospective or randomized trial has demonstrated that higher doses than the standard FDA-approved dose of vancomycin will result in better outcome for MRSA VAP. The presence of an *agr* II polymorphism in MRSA isolates may result in failure, no matter what the dose of vancomycin (69).

An alternative treatment strategy is to look for synergism. Concomitant rifampin or aminoglycosides have not been studied in pneumonia cases but anecdotally have not improved outcome. Compassionate use of quinupristin/dalfopristin plus vancomycin eradicated infection in five patients who had failed glycopeptide monotherapy for non-vancomycin-intermediate *S. aureus* (VISA) non-pneumonic MRSA infection (70).

The response to vancomycin, at least with the standard dose of 2 g/day, is clearly not ideal. Alternative agents have therefore been studied and introduced into clinical practice.

Linezolid

Linezolid is the first of a new class of antibiotics called oxazolidones, whose unique mechanism of action interferes with the assembly of the initiation complex for protein translation by binding to the ribosomal 50S subunit (55,72–73). Linezolid was compared to vancomycin in two double-blinded, randomized controlled trials for the treatment of suspected gram-positive nosocomial pneumonia (25,61). The first study of 402 patients demonstrated equivalent clinical outcomes between the linezolid and vancomycin groups, with clinical cure rates of 66% and 68%, respectively (61). Unfortunately, only a limited number of patients with MRSA pneumonia were enrolled (only nine patients in the vancomycin group). However, the FDA released linezolid for treatment of suspected gram-positive nosocomial pneumonia based on this trial.

The second larger trial enrolled an additional 623 patients with nosocomial pneumonia, with a larger number of MRSA cases (25). Although no significant clinical outcome difference was demonstrated in the entire population, the subgroup of MRSA pneumonia patients had 20% better clinical cure rates with linezolid than those treated with vancomycin. The survival rate was also greater in the subset of patients with APACHE-II scores of 16 to 19 treated with linezolid.

Data from the subset of patients with MRSA pneumonia from both studies were combined for analysis (74). Significantly higher clinical cure rates were found with linezolid than with vancomycin (59% vs. 35%).

Logistic regression analysis confirmed linezolid therapy as a significant predictor of clinical cure in MRSA nosocomial pneumonia, along with single-lobe pneumonia, absence of oncologic and renal comorbidities, and absence of VAP. Logistic regression analysis specifically of MRSA VAP confirmed that linezolid treatment remained a significant predictor of clinical cure. The rates for clinical cure were 62% for linezolid versus 21% for vancomycin ($P = 0.001$) (75). Outcome in VAP confirmed by invasive procedures or blood cultures followed the same pattern as the overall group. Most significant was documentation of a significant survival benefit of linezolid over vancomycin (85% vs. 67%) (74).

Several reasons for the superior response to linezolid are possible. Linezolid has a high volume of distribution and penetrates well into tissue (76). Steady-state levels in uninfected patients showed mean linezolid levels in BAL and alveolar macrophages were 25.09 and 8.10 mg/L, respectively (77). In another cohort of healthy volunteers, steady-state BAL levels were four times greater than serum levels at all time points after dosing (78). The concentration of linezolid in epithelial lining fluid (ELF) remained above the MIC for *S. aureus* 100% of the time during the 12-hour dosing interval and out to 24 hours after the last dose. Data from patients with suspected VAP found BAL/serum ratios were closer to one, although a nonstandardized nonbronchoscopic BAL technique was used (79).

For CA-MRSA pneumonia, no randomized clinical trials specifically address the antibiotic choice in this group. Recommendations for CA-MRSA CAP have followed the current standard of vancomycin treatment for MRSA VAP, in which clinical response and bacterial eradication remain poor. Linezolid, because of its mechanism of action, interferes with toxin production (80), whereas vancomycin and teicoplanin do not (81). This factor may be critical when necrotizing pneumonia is present.

None of the main adverse side effects of linezolid, which include neuropathy (optic and peripheral), myelosuppression, and potential monoamine oxidase inhibition, were seen in the clinical trial for pneumonia.

Thrombocytopenia, the easiest adverse response to detect, was comparable to that of vancomycin (82). Most adverse effects associated with linezolid require a longer exposure than the recommended seven- to eight-day treatment for VAP.

Other Therapy

The recent CA-MRSA outbreaks have stimulated interest in older drugs with in vitro susceptibility, such as minocycline and trimethoprim-sulfamethoxazole (72). Levaquin and moxifloxacin appear to be effective against CA-MRSA skin infections. None of these agents has been studied in either CA-MRSA or HA-MRSA pneumonia. Concern about rapid development of resistance exists (83).

Quinupristin/dalfopristin was compared to vancomycin in a prospective, randomized, multicenter trial in patients with gram-positive nosocomial pneumonia (60). While overall clinical success rates were equivalent, outcome in the subpopulation with MRSA was even worse than with vancomycin. In a small observational study, treatment of vancomycin-unresponsive MRSA infections (half pneumonia) with quinupristin-dalfopristin eradicated infection in 8 of 12 patients but only seven survived (84). This overall lack of efficacy and a significant adverse effect profile, including myalgias, arthralgias, and thrombophlebitis, limit its use for VAP.

Similarly, daptomycin, a promising new cyclic lipopeptide class of antibiotic with the unique property of promoting efflux of potassium out of bacterial cells, was found to be inferior to a cephalosporin for CAP (72,85). The inability of daptomycin, with its large molecular size, to adequately treat pneumonia may be due to poor penetration into lung tissue (86). Daptomycin also has a significant adverse effect profile with a risk of rhabdomyolysis, especially with concomitant statins (72,85).

Tigecycline, the first member of the glycylcycline class of antibiotics (analogs of tetracycline), has already been released for complicated skin and intra-abdominal infections (72,87). Data on activity for MRSA pneumonia are pending.

A variety of new antibiotics with activity against MRSA are being evaluated. New glycopeptides with prolonged half-lives are also being studied, but no human clinical data is yet available. These include oritavancin (72,88), dalbavancin (72,88), and telavancin (TD-6424) (89,90). Also, in development are cephalosporins and carbapenems with activity against MRSA.

PREVENTION STRATEGIES

General

General VAP prevention strategies apply to prevention of MRSA VAP as well. Avoidance of intubation in the first place with selective use of noninvasive ventilation, sedation holidays and protocolized weaning strategies, elevating the head of the bed, and appropriate infection control strategies are all important (23). Use of accurate diagnostic strategies to avoid excessive or unneeded antibiotics can also decrease the incidence of MRSA pneumonia, at least as measured by a decrease in the overall use of glycopeptides (91).

Prevention of CA-MRSA outbreaks is based on education of healthcare providers and adherence to basic infection control principles. Limited data from correctional facilities, military recruits, and competitive sports participants suggest that basic personal and environmental hygiene interventions are effective in controlling outbreaks (43,44,92).

Decreasing *Staphylococcus aureus* Colonization

The only aspect of prevention of MRSA VAP is addressing nasal and subsequent oropharyngeal colonization with *S. aureus*. Mupirocin has been recommended for clearance of nasal MRSA carriage during outbreaks (55). In a nonepidemic setting, eradication of MRSA nasal carriage with mupirocin ranged from 44% to 100%, but extranasal eradication was poor (93,94). No MRSA isolates developed high level mupirocin resistance.

Selective decontamination of the digestive (SDD) tract decreases mortality and the risk of pneumonia and bacteremia (95,96). While SDD seems to decrease the rates of MDR gram-negative bacteria, its effect on MRSA is conflicting (97–101). Topical vancomycin gel in the oropharynx alone significantly reduced the incidence of MRSA VAP without increasing the incidence of vancomycin-resistant organisms (102–104). The long-term effects of antibiotic prophylaxis to decrease MRSA colonization remain unclear.

CONCLUSIONS

Pneumonias, both HAP and CAP, due to MRSA pose significant management problems. Risk factors can be identified, and prevention strategies try to modify some of these factors when possible. Current data suggests that linezolid is a superior treatment choice for MRSA VAP in terms of pulmonary penetration and clinical efficacy. No study specifically addresses treatment of CA-MRSA CAP, so treatment is based on extrapolation from the HAP data and the ability of CA-MRSA to produce a toxin. Regardless, judicious use of appropriate antibiotics is crucial not only in the effective treatment of MDR pneumonias but also in the prevention of future complications.

REFERENCES

1. Saravolatz LD, Markowitz N, Arking L, Pohlod D, Fisher E. Methicillin-resistant *Staphylococcus aureus*. Epidemiologic observations during a community-acquired outbreak. Ann Intern Med 1982; 96:11–16.
2. Panton PN, Valentine FCO. Staphylococcal toxin. Lancet 1931; 1:506–508.
3. Lindsay JA, Holden MT. *Staphylococcus aureus*: superbug, super genome? Trends Microbiol 2004; 12:378–385.
4. Lina G, Piemont Y, Godail-Gamot F, et al. Involvement of Panton-Valentine leukocidin-producing *Staphylococcus aureus* in primary skin infections and pneumonia. Clin Infect Dis 1999; 29:1128–1132.

5. Naimi TS, LeDell KH, Como-Sabetti K, et al. Comparison of community- and health care-associated methicillin-resistant *Staphylococcus aureus* infection. J Am Med Assoc 2003; 290:2976–2984.

6. Francis JS, Doherty MC, Lopatin U, et al. Severe community-onset pneumonia in healthy adults caused by methicillin-resistant *Staphylococcus aureus* carrying the Panton-Valentine leukocidin genes. Clin Infect Dis 2005; 40:100–107.

7. Vandenesch F, Naimi T, Enright MC, et al. Community-acquired methicillin-resistant *Staphylococcus aureus* carrying Panton-Valentine leukocidin genes: worldwide emergence. Emerg Infect Dis 2003; 9:978–984.

8. Gillet Y, Issartel B, Vanhems P, et al. Association between *Staphylococcus aureus* strains carrying gene for Panton-Valentine leukocidin and highly lethal necrotising pneumonia in young immunocompetent patients. Lancet 2002; 359:753–759.

9. Ellis MW, Hospenthal DR, Dooley DP, Gray PJ, Murray CK. Natural history of community-acquired methicillin-resistant *Staphylococcus aureus* colonization and infection in soldiers. Clin Infect Dis 2004; 39:971–979.

10. Hageman JC, Uyeki TM, Francis JS, et al. Severe community-acquired pneumonia due to *Staphylococcus aureus*, 2003–04 influenza season. Emerg Infect Dis 2006; 12:894–899.

11. McGahee W, Lowy FD. Staphylococcal infections in the intensive care unit. Semin Respir Infect 2000; 15:308–313.

12. Noskin GA, Rubin RJ, Schentag JJ, et al. The burden of *Staphylococcus aureus* infections on hospitals in the United States: an analysis of the 2000 and 2001 Nationwide Inpatient Sample Database. Arch Intern Med 2005; 165:1756–1761.

13. Hubmayr RD, Burchardi H, Elliot M, et al. Statement of the 4th international consensus conference in critical care on ICU-acquired pneumonia—Chicago, Illinois, May 2002. Intensive Care Med 2002; 28:1521–1536.

14. Fridkin SK. Increasing prevalence of antimicrobial resistance in intensive care units. Crit Care Med 2001; 29:N64–N68.

15. Fagon JY, Chastre J, Hance AJ, Montravers P, Novara A, Gibert C. Nosocomial pneumonia in ventilated patients: a cohort study evaluating attributable mortality and hospital stay. Am J Med 1993; 94:281–288.

16. Heyland DK, Cook DJ, Griffith L, Keenan SP, Brun-Buisson C. The attributable morbidity and mortality of ventilator-associated pneumonia in the critically ill patient. The Canadian critical trials group. Am J Respir Crit Care Med 1999; 159:1249–1256.

17. Torres A, Carlet J. Ventilator-associated pneumonia. European task force on ventilator-associated pneumonia. Eur Respir J 2001; 17:1034–1045.

18. Trouillet JL, Chastre J, Vuagnat A, et al. Ventilator-associated pneumonia caused by potentially drug-resistant bacteria. Am J Respir Crit Care Med 1998; 157:531–539.

19. Rello J, Sa-Borges M, Correa H, Leal SR, Baraibar J. Variations in etiology of ventilator-associated pneumonia across four treatment sites: implications for antimicrobial prescribing practices. Am J Respir Crit Care Med 1999; 160:608–613.

20. Babcock HM, Zack JE, Garrison T, Trovillion E, Kollef MH, Fraser VJ. Ventilator-associated pneumonia in a multi-hospital system: differences in microbiology by location. Infect Control Hosp Epidemiol 2003; 24: 853–858.

21. Namias N, Samiian L, Nino D, et al. Incidence and susceptibility of pathogenic bacteria vary between intensive care units within a single hospital: implications for empiric antibiotic strategies. J Trauma 2000; 49:638–645; discussion 645–646.

22. Ibrahim EH, Ward S, Sherman G, Schaiff R, Fraser VJ, Kollef MH. Experience with a clinical guideline for the treatment of ventilator-associated pneumonia. Crit Care Med 2001; 29:1109–1115.

23. Guidelines for the management of adults with hospital-acquired, ventilator-associated, and healthcare-associated pneumonia. Am J Respir Crit Care Med 2005; 171:388–416.

24. Fagon JY, Chastre J, Domart Y, et al. Nosocomial pneumonia in patients receiving continuous mechanical ventilation. Prospective analysis of 52 episodes with use of a protected specimen brush and quantitative culture techniques. Am Rev Respir Dis 1989; 139:877–884.

25. Wunderink RG, Cammarata SK, Oliphant TH, Kollef MH. Continuation of a randomized, double-blind, multicenter study of linezolid versus vancomycin in the treatment of patients with nosocomial pneumonia. Clin Ther 2003; 25:980–992.

26. Rello J, Sole-Violan J, Sa-Borges M, et al. Pneumonia caused by oxacillin-resistant *Staphylococcus aureus* treated with glycopeptides. Crit Care Med 2005; 33:1983–1987.

27. Rello J, Torres A, Ricart M, et al. Ventilator-associated pneumonia by *Staphylococcus aureus*. Comparison of methicillin-resistant and methicillin-sensitive episodes. Am J Respir Crit Care Med 1994; 150:1545–1549.

28. Gonzalez C, Rubio M, Romero-Vivas J, Gonzalez M, Picazo JJ. Bacteremic pneumonia due to *Staphylococcus aureus*: a comparison of disease caused by methicillin-resistant and methicillin-susceptible organisms. Clin Infect Dis 1999; 29:1171–1177.

29. Cosgrove SE, Sakoulas G, Perencevich EN, Schwaber MJ, Karchmer AW, Carmeli Y. Comparison of mortality associated with methicillin-resistant and methicillin-susceptible *Staphylococcus aureus* bacteremia: a meta-analysis. Clin Infect Dis 2003; 36:53–59.

30. Shorr AF, Tabak YP, Gupta V, Johannes R, Liu LZ, Kollef MH. Morbidity and cost burden of methicillin-resistant *Staphylococcus aureus* in early onset ventilator-associated pneumonia. Crit Care 2006; 10:R97.

31. Foster TJ. The *Staphylococcus aureus* "superbug." J Clin Invest 2004; 114:1693–1696.

32. Sanford MD, Widmer AF, Bale MJ, Jones RN, Wenzel RP. Efficient detection and long-term persistence of the carriage of methicillin-resistant *Staphylococcus aureus*. Clin Infect Dis 1994; 19:1123–1128.

33. Huang SS, Platt R. Risk of methicillin-resistant *Staphylococcus aureus* infection after previous infection or colonization. Clin Infect Dis 2003; 36:281–285.

34. Garrouste-Orgeas M, Timsit JF, Kallel H, et al. Colonization with methicillin-resistant *Staphylococcus aureus* in ICU patients: morbidity, mortality, and glycopeptide use. Infect Control Hosp Epidemiol 2001; 22:687–692.

35. Deryke CA, Lodise TP Jr, Rybak MJ, McKinnon PS. Epidemiology, treatment, and outcomes of nosocomial bacteremic *Staphylococcus aureus* pneumonia. Chest 2005; 128:1414–1422.

36. MacDougall C, Powell JP, Johnson CK, Edmond MB, Polk RE. Hospital and community fluoroquinolone use and resistance in *Staphylococcus aureus* and *Escherichia coli* in 17 US hospitals. Clin Infect Dis 2005; 41:435–440.

37. Monnet DL, MacKenzie FM, Lopez-Lozano JM, et al. Antimicrobial drug use and methicillin-resistant *Staphylococcus aureus*, Aberdeen, 1996–2000. Emerg Infect Dis 2004; 10:1432–1441.

38. El-Solh AA, Pietrantoni C, Bhat A, et al. Microbiology of severe aspiration pneumonia in institutionalized elderly. Am J Respir Crit Care Med 2003; 167:1650–1654.

39. Drinka PJ, Gauerke C, Le D. Antimicrobial use and methicillin-resistant *Staphylococcus aureus* in a large nursing home. J Am Med Dir Assoc 2004; 5:256–258.

40. Mendelson G, Yearmack Y, Granot E, Ben-Israel J, Colodner R, Raz R. *Staphylococcus aureus* carrier state among elderly residents of a long-term care facility. J Am Med Dir Assoc 2003; 4:125–127.

41. Pujol M, Corbella X, Pena C, et al. Clinical and epidemiological findings in mechanically-ventilated patients with methicillin-resistant *Staphylococcus aureus* pneumonia. Eur J Clin Microbiol Infect Dis 1998; 17:622–628.

42. Ho PL. Carriage of methicillin-resistant *Staphylococcus aureus*, ceftazidime-resistant Gram-negative bacilli, and vancomycin-resistant enterococci before and after intensive care unit admission. Crit Care Med 2003; 31:1175–1182.

43. Methicillin-resistant *Staphylococcus aureus* infections in correctional facilities—Georgia, California, and Texas, 2001–2003. Morb Mortal Wkly Rep 2003; 52:992–996.

44. Zinderman CE, Conner B, Malakooti MA, LaMar JE, Armstrong A, Bohnker BK. Community-acquired methicillin-resistant *Staphylococcus aureus* among military recruits. Emerg Infect Dis 2004; 10:941–944.

45. Oztoprak N, Cevik MA, Akinci E, et al. Risk factors for ICU-acquired methicillin-resistant *Staphylococcus aureus* infections. Am J Infect Control 2006; 34:1–5.

46. Lucet JC, Paoletti X, Lolom I, et al. Successful long-term program for controlling methicillin-resistant *Staphylococcus aureus* in intensive care units. Intensive Care Med 2005; 31:1051–1057.

47. Hsieh AH, Bishop MJ, Kubilis PS, Newell DW, Pierson DJ. Pneumonia following closed head injury. Am Rev Respir Dis 1992; 146:290–294.

48. Rello J, Ausina V, Ricart M, Puzo C, Net A, Prats G. Nosocomial pneumonia in critically ill comatose patients: need for a differential therapeutic approach. Eur Respir J 1992; 5:1249–1253.

49. Berrouane Y, Daudenthun I, Riegel B, et al. Early onset pneumonia in neurosurgical intensive care unit patients. J Hosp Infect 1998; 40:275–280.

50. Bronchard R, Albaladejo P, Brezac G, et al. Early onset pneumonia: risk factors and consequences in head trauma patients. Anesthesiology 2004; 100:234–239.

51. Campbell W, Hendrix E, Schwalbe R, Fattom A, Edelman R. Head-injured patients who are nasal carriers of *Staphylococcus aureus* are at high risk for *Staphylococcus aureus* pneumonia. Crit Care Med 1999; 27:798–801.

52. Ewig S, Torres A, El-Ebiary M, et al. Bacterial colonization patterns in mechanically ventilated patients with traumatic and medical head injury. Incidence, risk factors, and association with ventilator-associated pneumonia. Am J Respir Crit Care Med 1999; 159:188–198.

53. Sirvent JM, Torres A, Vidaur L, Armengol J, de Batlle J, Bonet A. Tracheal colonisation within 24 hr of intubation in patients with head trauma: risk factor for developing early-onset ventilator-associated pneumonia. Intensive Care Med 2000; 26:1369–1372.

54. Bassetti S, Bischoff WE, Walter M, et al. Dispersal of *Staphylococcus aureus* into the air associated with a rhinovirus infection. Infect Control Hosp Epidemiol 2005; 26:196–203.

55. Chambers HF. Methicillin resistance in staphylococci: molecular and biochemical basis and clinical implications. Clin Microbiol Rev 1997; 10:781–791.

56. Lowy FD. *Staphylococcus aureus* infections. N Engl J Med 1998; 339:520–532.

57. Levine DP, Fromm BS, Reddy BR. Slow response to vancomycin or vancomycin plus rifampin in methicillin-resistant *Staphylococcus aureus* endocarditis. Ann Intern Med 1991; 115:674–680.

58. Moise-Broder PA, Forrest A, Birmingham MC, Schentag JJ. Pharmacodynamics of vancomycin and other antimicrobials in patients with *Staphylococcus aureus* lower respiratory tract infections. Clin Pharmacokinet 2004; 43:925–942.

59. Moise PA, Forrest A, Birmingham MC, Schentag JJ. The efficacy and safety of linezolid as treatment for *Staphylococcus aureus* infections in compassionate use patients who are intolerant of, or who have failed to respond to, vancomycin. J Antimicrob Chemother 2002; 50:1017–1026.

60. Fagon J, Patrick H, Haas DW, et al. Treatment of gram-positive nosocomial pneumonia. Prospective randomized comparison of quinupristin/dalfopristin versus vancomycin. Nosocomial Pneumonia Group. Am J Respir Crit Care Med 2000; 161:753–762.

61. Rubinstein E, Cammarata S, Oliphant T, Wunderink R. Linezolid (PNU-100766) versus vancomycin in the treatment of hospitalized patients with nosocomial pneumonia: a randomized, double-blind, multicenter study. Clin Infect Dis 2001; 32:402–412.

62. Baughman RP, Kerr MA. Ventilator-associated pneumonia patients who do not reduce bacteria from the lungs have a worse prognosis. J Intensive Care Med 2003; 18:269–274.

63. Cruciani M, Gatti G, Lazzarini L, et al. Penetration of vancomycin into human lung tissue. J Antimicrob Chemother 1996; 38:865–869.

64. Lamer C, de Beco V, Soler P, et al. Analysis of vancomycin entry into pulmonary lining fluid by bronchoalveolar lavage in critically ill patients. Antimicrob Agents Chemother 1993; 37:281–286.

65. Georges H, Leroy O, Alfandari S, et al. Pulmonary disposition of vancomycin in critically ill patients. Eur J Clin Microbiol Infect Dis 1997; 16:385–388.

66. Moise PA, Forrest A, Bhavnani SM, Birmingham MC, Schentag JJ. Area under the inhibitory curve and a pneumonia scoring system for predicting outcomes of vancomycin therapy for respiratory infections by *Staphylococcus aureus*. Am J Health Syst Pharm 2000; 57(suppl 2):S4–S9.

67. Sakoulas G, Moise-Broder PA, Schentag J, Forrest A, Moellering RC Jr, Eliopoulos GM. Relationship of MIC and bactericidal activity to efficacy of vancomycin for treatment of methicillin-resistant *Staphylococcus aureus* bacteremia. J Clin Microbiol 2004; 42:2398–2402.

68. Wysocki M, Delatour F, Faurisson F, et al. Continuous versus intermittent infusion of vancomycin in severe Staphylococcal infections: prospective multicenter randomized study. Antimicrob Agents Chemother 2001; 45:2460–2467.

69. Moise-Broder PA, Sakoulas G, Eliopoulos GM, Schentag JJ, Forrest A, Moellering RC Jr. Accessory gene regulator group II polymorphism in methicillin-resistant *Staphylococcus aureus* is predictive of failure of vancomycin therapy. Clin Infect Dis 2004; 38:1700–1705.

70. Cepeda JA, Whitehouse T, Cooper B, et al. Linezolid versus teicoplanin in the treatment of Gram-positive infections in the critically ill: a randomized, double-blind, multicentre study. J Antimicrob Chemother 2004; 53:345–355.

71. Sgarabotto D, Cusinato R, Narne E, et al. Synercid plus vancomycin for the treatment of severe methicillin-resistant *Staphylococcus aureus* and coagulase-negative staphylococci infections: evaluation of 5 cases. Scand J Infect Dis 2002; 34:122–126.

72. Anstead GM, Owens AD. Recent advances in the treatment of infections due to resistant *Staphylococcus aureus*. Curr Opin Infect Dis 2004; 17:549–555.

73. Eliopoulos GM. Quinupristin-dalfopristin and linezolid: evidence and opinion. Clin Infect Dis 2003; 36:473–481.

74. Wunderink RG, Rello J, Cammarata SK, Croos-Dabrera RV, Kollef MH. Linezolid vs vancomycin: analysis of two double-blind studies of patients with methicillin-resistant *Staphylococcus aureus* nosocomial pneumonia. Chest 2003; 124:1789–1797.

75. Kollef MH, Rello J, Cammarata SK, Croos-Dabrera RV, Wunderink RG. Clinical cure and survival in Gram-positive ventilator-associated pneumonia: retrospective analysis of two double-blind studies comparing linezolid with vancomycin. Intensive Care Med 2004; 30:388–394.

76. Gee T, Ellis R, Marshall G, Andrews J, Ashby J, Wise R. Pharmacokinetics and tissue penetration of linezolid following multiple oral doses. Antimicrob Agents Chemother 2001; 45:1843–1846.

77. Honeybourne D, Tobin C, Jevons G, Andrews J, Wise R. Intrapulmonary penetration of linezolid. J Antimicrob Chemother 2003; 51:1431–1434.

78. Conte JE Jr, Golden JA, Kipps J, Zurlinden E. Intrapulmonary pharmacokinetics of linezolid. Antimicrob Agents Chemother 2002; 46:1475–1480.

79. Boselli E, Breilh D, Rimmele T, et al. Pharmacokinetics and intrapulmonary concentrations of linezolid administered to critically ill patients with ventilator-associated pneumonia. Crit Care Med 2005; 33:1529–1533.
80. Bernardo K, Pakulat N, Fleer S, et al. Subinhibitory concentrations of linezolid reduce *Staphylococcus aureus* virulence factor expression. Antimicrob Agents Chemother 2004; 48:546–555.
81. Ohlsen K, Ziebuhr W, Koller KP, Hell W, Wichelhaus TA, Hacker J. Effects of subinhibitory concentrations of antibiotics on alpha-toxin (*hla*) gene expression of methicillin-sensitive and methicillin-resistant *Staphylococcus aureus* isolates. Antimicrob Agents Chemother 1998; 42:2817–2823.
82. Nasraway SA, Shorr AF, Kuter DJ, O'Grady N, Le VH, Cammarata SK. Linezolid does not increase the risk of thrombocytopenia in patients with nosocomial pneumonia: comparative analysis of linezolid and vancomycin use. Clin Infect Dis 2003; 37:1609–1616.
83. Shopsin B, Zhao X, Kreiswirth BN, Tillotson GS, Drlica K. Are the new quinolones appropriate treatment for community-acquired methicillin-resistant *Staphylococcus aureus*? Int J Antimicrob Agents 2004; 24:32–34.
84. Sander A, Beiderlinden M, Schmid EN, Peters J. Clinical experience with quinupristin-dalfopristin as rescue treatment of critically ill patients infected with methicillin-resistant staphylococci. Intensive Care Med 2002; 28:1157–1160.
85. Fenton C, Keating GM, Curran MP. Daptomycin. Drugs 2004; 64:445–455; discussion 457–458.
86. Carpenter CF, Chambers HF. Daptomycin: another novel agent for treating infections due to drug-resistant gram-positive pathogens. Clin Infect Dis 2004; 38:994–1000.
87. Zhanel GG, Homenuik K, Nichol K, et al. The glycylcyclines: a comparative review with the tetracyclines. Drugs 2004; 64:63–88.
88. Van Bambeke F, Van Laethem Y, Courvalin P, Tulkens PM. Glycopeptide antibiotics: from conventional molecules to new derivatives. Drugs 2004; 64:913–936.
89. Goldstein EJ, Citron DM, Merriam CV, Warren YA, Tyrrell KL, Fernandez HT. In vitro activities of the new semisynthetic glycopeptide telavancin (TD-6424), vancomycin, daptomycin, linezolid, and four comparator agents against anaerobic gram-positive species and *Corynebacterium* spp. Antimicrob Agents Chemother 2004; 48:2149–2152.
90. Reyes N, Skinner R, Kaniga K, et al. Efficacy of telavancin (TD-6424), a rapidly bactericidal lipoglycopeptide with multiple mechanisms of action,

in a murine model of pneumonia induced by methicillin-resistant *Staphylococcus aureus*. Antimicrob Agents Chemother 2005; 49:4344–4346.

91. Fagon JY, Chastre J, Wolff M, et al. Invasive and noninvasive strategies for management of suspected ventilator-associated pneumonia. A randomized trial. Ann Intern Med 2000; 132:621–630.

92. Methicillin-resistant *Staphylococcus aureus* infections among competitive sports participants—Colorado, Indiana, Pennsylvania, and Los Angeles County, 2000–2003. Morb Mortal Wkly Rep 2003; 52:793–795.

93. Harbarth S, Dharan S, Liassine N, Herrault P, Auckenthaler R, Pittet D. Randomized, placebo-controlled, double-blind trial to evaluate the efficacy of mupirocin for eradicating carriage of methicillin-resistant *Staphylococcus aureus*. Antimicrob Agents Chemother 1999; 43:1412–1416.

94. Parras F, Guerrero MC, Bouza E, et al. Comparative study of mupirocin and oral co-trimoxazole plus topical fusidic acid in eradication of nasal carriage of methicillin-resistant *Staphylococcus aureus*. Antimicrob Agents Chemother 1995; 39:175–179.

95. Krueger WA, Lenhart FP, Neeser G, et al. Influence of combined intravenous and topical antibiotic prophylaxis on the incidence of infections, organ dysfunctions, and mortality in critically ill surgical patients: a prospective, stratified, randomized, double-blind, placebo-controlled clinical trial. Am J Respir Crit Care Med 2002; 166:1029–1037.

96. de Jonge E, Schultz MJ, Spanjaard L, et al. Effects of selective decontamination of digestive tract on mortality and acquisition of resistant bacteria in intensive care: a randomised controlled trial. Lancet 2003; 362:1011–1016.

97. de Jonge E. Effects of selective decontamination of digestive tract on mortality and antibiotic resistance in the intensive-care unit. Curr Opin Crit Care 2005; 11:144–149.

98. Verwaest C, Verhaegen J, Ferdinande P, et al. Randomized, controlled trial of selective digestive decontamination in 600 mechanically ventilated patients in a multidisciplinary intensive care unit. Crit Care Med 1997; 25:63–71.

99. Leone M, Albanese J, Antonini F, Nguyen-Michel A, Martin C. Long-term (6-year) effect of selective digestive decontamination on antimicrobial resistance in intensive care, multiple-trauma patients. Crit Care Med 2003; 31:2090–2095.

100. Lingnau W, Berger J, Javorsky F, Fille M, Allerberger F, Benzer H. Changing bacterial ecology during a five-year period of selective intestinal decontamination. J Hosp Infect 1998; 39:195–206.

101. Silvestri L, Milanese M, Oblach L, et al. Enteral vancomycin to control methicillin-resistant *Staphylococcus aureus* outbreak in mechanically ventilated patients. Am J Infect Control 2002; 30:391–399.
102. Bergmans DC, Bonten MJ, Gaillard CA, et al. Prevention of ventilator-associated pneumonia by oral decontamination: a prospective, randomized, double-blind, placebo-controlled study. Am J Respir Crit Care Med 2001; 164:382–388.
103. Pugin J, Auckenthaler R, Lew DP, Suter PM. Oropharyngeal decontamination decreases incidence of ventilator-associated pneumonia. A randomized, placebo-controlled, double-blind clinical trial. J Am Med Assoc 1991; 265:2704–2710.
104. Silvestri L, van Saene HK, Milanese M, et al. Prevention of MRSA pneumonia by oral vancomycin decontamination: a randomised trial. Eur Respir J 2004; 23:921–926.

Central Venous Access and MRSA Bacteremia

8

Renae E. Stafford
Department of Surgery, University of North Carolina,
Chapel Hill, North Carolina, U.S.A.

INTRODUCTION

Central venous catheters (CVCs) are used in the healthcare setting for the administration of intravenous (IV) fluids, blood, and medications and for hemodynamic monitoring. Catheter-related bloodstream infections (CR-BSI), are bloodstream infections associated with venous access devices, are the most common type of nosocomial bloodstream infection (1). Some 250,000 CR-BSI have been estimated to occur each year (2). They are most commonly associated with the use of a CVC and are a major cause of morbidity and mortality (1,3). Because of the morbidity, mortality, and cost associated with CR-BSI, the clinician must have a working understanding of the epidemiology, diagnosis, and management of these common nosocomial infections.

EPIDEMIOLOGY

CR-BSI associated with CVCs are most commonly related to nontunneled CVCs, but are also seen in patients with tunneled catheters. CVC use in the intensive care unit is associated with an increased incidence of infection, secondary to use for extended periods of time, multiple manipulations of the catheter, and a greater potential for being colonized with hospital-acquired organisms (3). The incidence of CVC bloodstream infections ranges from 8.5 to 19.8 infections per 1000 catheter days, with an average rate of 5.3 per 1000 catheter days (3,4). Pathogenesis of these infections is related to extraluminal colonization from the skin, seeding from hematogenous spread and intraluminal colonization of the catheter (5). The presence of multiple lumens in a single CVC is associated with an increased risk of CR-BSI (6,7) and each lumen is a potential source for infection (8).

The most common causative organisms that cause CR-BSI are gram-positive bacteria such as Staphylococcal organisms, including coagulase-negative *Staphylococcus* and coagulase-positive *Staphylococcus aureus* and *Enterococcus* (1,9). Methicillin-resistant *S. aureus* (MRSA) is now the most common cause of nosocomial- or hospital-acquired infection, and it accounts for approximately 55% of all *Staphylococcus* isolates (1). Risk factors for MRSA infection include recent exposure to a healthcare setting, indwelling catheters, residence in a long-term care facility, presence of an open wound, and previous exposure to antibiotics (1,10–12).

MRSA bacteremia is associated with tunneled and nontunneled CVCs, and it is suggested that it may be more commonly seen in patients with tunneled CVCs such as those used for hemodialysis (13,14). It is also found to be the most common organism causing bloodstream infection after liver transplantation (15). MRSA-associated infections such as bacteremia are associated with increased morbidity and mortality when compared to methicillin-sensitive staphylococcal infections (16–19). The presence of MRSA CR-BSI is associated with a risk ratio of 2.09 for the development of hematogenous complications, which might explain a higher cost and mortality. In one study, 23% of MRSA bacteremias were found to be catheter-related with an attributable mortality for MRSA bacteremia of 23.4% compared to a 1.3% attributable mortality for methicillin-sensitive *S. aureus* (MSSA) bacteremia (18). MRSA CR-BSI is also associated with higher median hospital costs (20).

DIAGNOSIS

The diagnosis of CR-BSI is suspected based on clinical signs and symptoms in a patient who has a CVC. These may include purulence or inflammation at the catheter site, fever, malaise, chills, and hypotension. However, the sensitivity and specificity of these factors is variable (5). An MRSA CR-BSI should be suspected in any patient with risk factors for MRSA and central venous access. A positive blood culture for MRSA, clinical signs and symptoms, and a CVC increase the suspicion for CR-BSI. The addition of a quantitative or semiquantitative culture of the CVC that yields the same organism as that obtained from peripheral blood cultures and the absence of any other identifiable source for infection confirms the diagnosis (5).

In the patient with erythema or purulent drainage from a CVC site, a gram stain may be helpful but it does not necessarily mean that there is a CR-BSI. It is recommended that two sets of blood cultures be obtained from a peripheral vein when possible, because a positive blood culture drawn from a CVC has a lower positive predictive value than that drawn from a peripheral site (5,21).

When two sets of blood cultures cannot be drawn peripherally, one may be drawn through the CVC and the quantitative culture results compared. If the quantitative bacterial colony count in the culture drawn through CVC is at least five times that for the peripheral culture, a CR-BSI is likely (5,22). If more than one lumen is present in the CVC, drawing a culture from each lumen will increase the sensitivity of the test (23), because sampling one lumen has only a 60% chance of detecting significant colonization (8).

When CVCs are removed and cultured, a positive result that yields the same organism as a blood culture helps to confirm the diagnosis. Semiquantitative or quantitative cultures of the catheter may be done depending on individual laboratory standards. Semiquantitative culture, as defined by Maki et al. (24), is obtained by rolling a portion of the catheter over an agar plate, incubation, and then counting of bacterial colonies. A yield of ≥ 15 colony-forming units (CFU) is considered positive. This is the most widely used method (5). Quantitative cultures are more labor-intensive, requiring serial dilutions and agar plating. A yield of $\geq 10^2$ CFU is considered positive for this method (5).

Finally, where quantitative blood cultures are not available, the differential time to positivity for CVC versus peripheral blood culture method may be helpful (5). This method compares the differential time to positivity for cultures drawn from CVC and a peripheral vein. This test is considered positive for a CR-BSI if the CVC culture is positive at least two hours earlier than one drawn peripherally. This time differential approach has a 91% sensitivity and a 94% specificity (25).

MANAGEMENT

The management of CR-BSI usually includes empiric IV antibiotic therapy directed at suspected organisms based on the clinical scenario, removal of the CVC or access device, and narrowing of the empiric antibiotic therapy based on culture and susceptibility results (Fig. 1). Management of complications of catheter-related bacteremia such as endocarditis, pneumonia, hematogenous seeding of other sites, and foreign bodies such as orthopedic hardware and pacemaker wires will depend on the complication involved. Both MSSA and MRSA may be associated with these complications.

In the patient who has a central venous access device and a suspected MRSA infection based on known risk factors, vancomycin, a bacteriostatic glycopeptide, is usually recommended as the first-line empiric antibiotic, because it has activity against MRSA in addition to the other common organisms that cause CR-BSI. However, vancomycin-resistant staphylococci have emerged (26). Alternative agents such as line-zolid, quinopristin/dalfopristin, daptomycin, and tigecycline could be used depending upon the patient's underlying disease and clinical scenario (5,27–30). Quinupristin-dalfopristin is a synthetic streptogramin combination agent with activity against MRSA. Daptomycin, a cyclic lipopeptide, is a bactericidal agent with MRSA activity. Linezolid is an agent that belongs to a class of drugs called oxazolidinones and has bacteriostatic activity against MRSA. Tigecycline belongs to the glycylcy-cline antibiotic class and is bactericidal. These agents are usually more

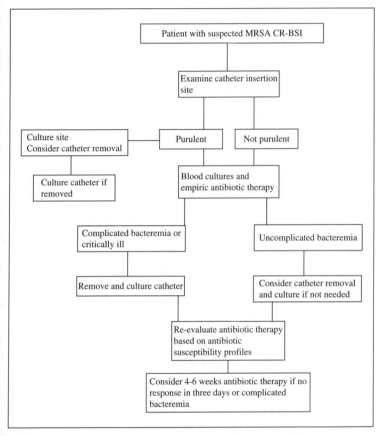

FIGURE 1   Management of patients with MRSA catheter-related bloodstream infection.

TABLE 1 Intravenous Antibiotics for Treatment of MRSA Catheter-Related Bloodstream Infections in Adults

Antibiotic	Initial dose	Adjust for renal insufficiency
Vancomycin	1 g IV q 12 hr[a]	Yes
Quinopristin–dalfopristin	7.5 mg/kg IV q 8 hr[a]	No
Linezolid	600 mg IV q 12 hr[a]	No
Tigecycline	100 mg IV then 50 mg q 12 hr[b]	No
Daptomycin	6 mg/kg IV q 24 hr[b]	Yes

[a]From Ref. 5, p. 1254.
[b]From Ref. 55.
Abbreviation: IV, intravenous.

costly, have differing side effect profiles, their use may be restricted by hospital formulary policies, and not all are Food and Drug Administration approved for bacteremia (Table 1). A promising investigational agent, dalbavancin, may be available in the future (4).

It is not clear whether the choice of an inappropriate empiric antibiotic or the timing of empiric therapy leads to an increase in mortality, but inappropriate empiric therapy has shown to be more likely in those patients with MRSA who have malignancy, no prior history of colonization with MRSA, and a long hospital stay prior to diagnosis (31,32). No matter what antibiotic agent is chosen initially, the susceptibility profile of the identified organism should be used to guide final therapy.

The duration of therapy for CVC-related bacteremia due to *S. aureus* and MRSA remains controversial, and there are no randomized trials that support a specific duration of therapy. Those patients with uncomplicated bacteremia with a good clinical response to treatment, such as rapid defervescence and decrease in WBC count, may be treated with 10 to 14 days of therapy. However, patients who are critically ill, fail to respond to antibiotic therapy (continued fever and elevated WBC or worsening of clinical status), or have persistent bacteremia should be re-evaluated. An undefined source of infection should be sought and antibiotic regimens should be re-evaluated. Patients with metastatic complications of their bacteremia, such as endocarditis, should be treated with a longer course of therapy (four to eight weeks) (5,33–35). It has been suggested that transesophageal echocardiography may be a cost-effective method to determine the duration of therapy in patients with uncomplicated staphylococcal bacteremia (36); however, others have found that this may not be necessary (35).

The removal of CVC, either by guidewire exchange or complete removal, in patients with suspected CR-BSI has long been a part of the management algorithm. Current guidelines for the patient with suspected CR-BSI include keeping the catheter in place while awaiting culture results in a patient with fever and mild to moderate disease, as the majority of these catheters, when cultured, will be sterile (5,37). Catheters are recommended to be removed for severe disease, erythema or purulence at the exit site, or for signs of unexplained sepsis.

Patients with tunneled catheters used for hemodialysis or chemotherapy, or who have implantable venous access devices, or have limited venous access options, present a challenge for the clinician. It is often not feasible to remove these devices initially, and the clinician must balance the likelihood of the catheter only being colonized versus being infected. In this setting, the catheter is often left in place and antibiotic therapy is initiated through the catheter. Additional antibiotic lock therapy may be used (5). This is performed by filling the catheter with pharmacologic concentrations of antibiotics and leaving them in the catheter for hours to days. Results from trials of catheter salvage with or without antibiotic lock therapy are variable.

Attempts at catheter salvage should be undertaken with caution. Failure to remove a catheter once *S. aureus* catheter-related bacteremia occurs is associated with an increased risk of hematogenous complications (19), and attempts at catheter salvage in hemodialysis patients is associated with epidural abscesses (38). In patients undergoing hemo-dialysis, catheter salvage was less likely to occur with gram-positive organism bacteremia, *S. aureus* most commonly, when compared to gram-negative bacteremia (39).

Failure to respond to appropriate antimicrobial therapy, persistent bacteremia, or the development of hematogenous complications should lead to an aggressive management strategy. If attempts at catheter salvage were made and appropriate antibiotics are being used, the CVC should be removed. Additionally, a search for other sites of infection such as orthopedic hardware and valvular vegetations should be undertaken.

PREVENTION

Given the significant morbidity, cost, and mortality associated with MRSA CR-BSI, today's medical practitioner must do whatever possible to prevent these infections. Strategies that have been proposed for prevention of CR-BSI include quality assurance and continuing education, selection of site of catheter insertion, hand hygiene and aseptic technique, use of antimicrobial/antiseptic impregnated catheters and cuffs, use of anti-biotic/antiseptic ointments at the insertion site, antibiotic lock prophy-laxis, scheduled replacement of nontunneled IV catheters and IV administration sets, avoiding multiple lumen catheters when possible, and use of needleless intravascular catheter systems (3).

Quality assurance and continuing education is shown to reduce the risk of CR-BSI (40). The site and technique of CVC placement is critical to prevention of CR-BSI. Placement of the CVC in the subclavian vein as opposed to the jugular vein is associated with a decreased risk of infection (41,42). Maximal barrier precautions that include hat, mask, sterile gown and gloves, and a large sterile field should be used (3,43). Aseptic technique using chlorhexidine gluconate-containing solutions, as opposed to povidine iodine for skin preparation, is associated with decreased risk of infection associated with gram-positive bacteria (44). The use of semipermeable transparent versus gauze dressings has been suggested as a risk factor for CR-BSI (41); however, this increased risk has not been demonstrated in a large meta-analysis (45). Either dressing is acceptable and should be changed when the dressing is moist or soiled, when a catheter is changed and according to individual institutional protocol (3,46).

Chlorhexidine/silver sulfadiazine-coated CVCs can reduce the risk of CR-BSI compared to noncoated standard catheters (47,48), but seems to be of benefit within the first two weeks of catheter placement (49). Antibiotic lock prophylaxis with vancomycin-containing solutions may be useful for preventing gram-positive bacteremia in neutropenic patients with long-term catheters (50,51), but routine use is not recommended due to potential for acquisition of vancomycin-resistant organisms such as *Enterococcus* (3).

Because an increased risk of CR-BSI is associated with multiple lumen CVCs, a determination of how much access is necessary should be made every time a CVC is placed and the CVC should have only the number of lumens that are necessary. Additionally, as soon as CVC use is no longer essential, the CVC should be removed as the risk of CR-BSI increases with the length of time the line is in place (7).

Scheduled replacement of CVCs by placement at a new site (52,53) or by guidewire exchange (54) is not associated with reduction in CR-BSI and is not recommended for functioning catheters with no evidence of local or systemic complications (3,7,46).

CONCLUSIONS

CR-BSIs are the most common type of nosocomial-acquired bloodstream infections. CR-BSI caused by MRSA accounts for an ever-increasing proportion of these infections and are associated with increased morbidity, mortality, and cost. Risk factors for MRSA CR-BSI include presence of a CVC, previous infection or colonization with MRSA, recent contact with the healthcare setting, residence in a long-term care facility, and previous exposure to antibiotics.

Management of these infections includes physical examination, empiric antibiotic therapy, culture of the CVC insertion site or catheter where appropriate, blood cultures, and refinement of antibiotic therapy based upon the antibiotic susceptibility profile of the organism. In certain clinical scenarios, the CVC may not need to be removed. Duration of therapy depends on the clinical status of the patient and presence or absence of hematogenous spread to other organs or indwelling devices. Management of hematogenous complications will depend on the complication that occurs. Prevention of these infections is the goal of a good infection control program.

REFERENCES

1. CDC. National Nosocomial Infections Surveillance (NNIS) System report. Report, data summary from January 1992–June 2003. Am J Infect Control 2003; 31:481–498.
2. Kluger DM, Maki DG. The relative risk of intravascular related bloodstream infections in adults (Abstract). In: Abstracts of the 39th Interscience Conference on Antimicrobial Agents and Chemotherapy. San Francisco, CA: American Society for Microbiology, 1999:514.
3. CDC. Guidelines for the prevention of intravascular catheter-related infections. MMWR 2002; 51:RR-10.
4. Raad I, Darouiche R, Vazquez J, et al. Efficacy and safety of weekly dalbavancin therapy for catheter-related bloodstream infection caused by gram-positive organisms. Clin Infect Dis 2005; 40:374–380.
5. Mermel LA, Farr BM, Sherertz RJ, et al. Guidelines for the management of intravascular catheter-related infections. Clin Infect Dis 2001; 32:1249–1272.
6. Dezfulian C, Lavelle J, Brahmajee BK, et al. Rates of infection for single-lumen versus multiple lumen central venous catheters: A meta-analysis. Crit Care Med 2003; 31:2385–2390.
7. Safdar N, Kluger DM, Maki DG. A review of risk factors for catheter-related bloodstream infection caused by percutaneously inserted, noncuffed central venous catheters. Implications for preventive strategies. Medicine 2002; 81:466–479.
8. Dobbins BM, Catton JA, Kite P, et al. Each lumen is a potential source of central venous catheter-related bloodstream infection. Crit Care Med 2003; 31:1688–1690.

9. Edmond MB, Wallace SE, McLish DK, et al. Nosocomial Bloodstream infections in United States hospitals: a three-year analysis. Clin Infect Dis 1999; 29:239–244.

10. Said-Salim B, Mathema B, Kreiswirth B. Community-acquired methicillin-resistant *Staphylococcus aureus*: An emerging pathogen. Infect Control Hosp Epidemiol 2003; 24:451–455.

11. Oztoprak N, Cevik MA, Akinci E, et al. Risk factors for hospital-acquired methicillin-resistant *Staphylococcus aureus* infection. Am J Infection 2006; 34:1–5.

12. Gonzalez C, Rubio M, Romero-Vivas, et al. Bacteremic pneumonia due to *Staphylococcus aureus*: A comparison of disease caused by methicillin-resistant and methicillin-susceptible organisms. Clin Infect Dis 1999; 29:1171–1177.

13. Rezende NA, Blumberg HM, Metzger BS, et al. Risk factors for methicillin-resistance among patients with *Staphylococcus aureus* bacteremia at the time of hospital admission. Am J Med Sci 2002; 323:117–123.

14. Reed SD, Friedman JY, Engemann JJ, et al. Costs and outcomes among hemodialysis-dependent patients with methicillin-resistant or methicillin-susceptible *Staphylococcus aureus* bacteremia. Infect Control Hosp Epidemiol 2005; 26:175–183.

15. Singh N, Gayowski T, Wagener MM, et al. Bloodstream infections in liver transplant recipients receiving tacrolimus. Clin Transplant 1997; 11:275–281.

16. Vincent JL, Sakr Y, Sprung CL, et al. Sepsis in European intensive care units: results of the SOAP study. Crit Care Med 2006; 34:344–353.

17. Taylor MD, Napolitano LM. Methicillin-resistant *Staphylococcus aureus* infections in vascular surgery: Increasing prevalence. Surg Infect 2004; 5:180–187.

18. Blot SI, Vandewoude KH, Hoste EA, et al. Outcome and attributable mortality in critically ill patients with bacteremia involving methicillin-susceptible and methicillin-resistant *Staphylococcus aureus*. Arch Intern Med 2002; 162:2229–2235.

19. Fowler VG, Justice A, Moore C, et al. Risk factors for hematogenous complications of intravascular catheter-associated *Staphylococcus aureus* bacteremia. Clin Infect Dis 2005; 40:695–703.

20. Kopp BJ, Nix DE, Armstrong EP. Clinical and economic analysis of methicillin-susceptible and -resistant *Staphylococcus aureus* infections. Ann Pharmacother 2004; 38:1377–1382.

21. DesJardin J. Clinical utility of blood cultures drawn from indwelling central venous catheters in hospitalized patients with cancer. Ann Intern Med 1999; 131:641–647.

22. Fan ST, Teoh-Chan CH, Lau KF. Evaluation of central venous catheter sepsis by differential quantitative blood culture. Eur J Clin Microbiol Infect Dis 1989; 8:142–144.

23. Catton JA, Dobbins BM, Kite P, et al. In situ diagnosis of intravascular catheter-related bloodstream infection: A comparison of quantitative culture, differential time to positivity, and endoluminal brushing. Crit Care Med 2005; 33:787–791.

24. Maki DG, Weise CE, Sarafin HW. A semiquantitative culture method for identifying intravenous catheter related infections. New Engl J Med 1977; 296:1305–1309.

25. Blot F, Schmidt E, Nitenberg G, et al. Earlier positivity of central venous versus peripheral blood cultures is highly predictive of catheter related sepsis. Eur J Clin Microbiol 1998; 36:105–109.

26. Chadwick P, Wooster S. Glycopeptide resistance in *Staphylococcus aureus*. J Infect 2000; 40:211–217.

27. Garcia R, Raad I. In vitro study of the potential role of quinuprisitn/dalfopristin in the treatment of catheter-related staphylococcal infections. Eur J Clin Microbiol Infect Dis 1996; 15:933–936.

28. Eliopolous GM. Quinupristin-dalfopristin and linezolid: Evidence and opinion. Cklin Infect Dis 2003; 36:473–481.

29. Seguti JA, Crank CW, Finney MS. Daptomycin for treatment of gram-positive bacteremia and infective endocarditis: A retrospective case series of 31 patients. Pharmacotherapy 2006; 26:347–352.

30. Lode H. Management of serious nosocomial bacterial infections: do current therapeutic options meet the need? Clin Microbiol Infect 2005; 11: 778–787.

31. Kim SH, Park WB, Lee CS, et al. Outcome of inappropriate empirical antibiotic therapy in patients with *Staphylococcus aureus* bacteremia: analytical strategy using propensity scores. Clin Microbiol Infect 2006; 12:13–21.

32. Fang CT, Shau WY, Hsueh PR, et al. Early empirical glycopeptide therapy for patients with methicillin-resistant *Staphylococcus aureus* bacteremia: impact on the outcome. J Antimicrob Chemother 2006; 57:511–519.

33. Malanoski GJ, Samore MH, Pefanis A, et al. *Staphylococcus aureus* catheter-associated bacteremia. Minimal effective therapy and unusual infectious complications associated with arterial sheath catheters. Arch Intern Med 1995; 155:1161–1166.

34. Zeylmaker MMP, Jaspers CA, van Kraaij MG, et al. Long-term infectious complications and their relation to treatment duration in catheter-related *Staphylococcus aureus* bacteremia. Eur J Clin Microbiol Infect Dis 2001; 20:380–384.

35. Pigrau C, Rodriguez D, Planes AM, et al. Management of catheter-related *Staphylococcus aureus* bacteremia: When may sonographic study be unnecessary? Eur J Clin Microbiol Infect Dis 2003; 22:713–719.

36. Rosen AB, Fowler VG, Corey GR, et al. Cost-effectiveness of transesophageal echocardiography to determine the duration of therapy for intravascular catheter-associated *Staphylococcus* bacteremia. Ann Intern Med 1999; 130:810–820.

37. O'Grady NP, Barie P, Bartlett J, et al. Practice parameters for evaluating new fever in critically ill adult patients. Crit Care Med 1998; 26: 392–408.

38. Kovalik EC, Raymond Jr, Albers FJ, et al. A clustering of epidural abscesses in chronic hemodialysis patients: risks of salvaging access catheters in cases of infection. J Am Soc Nephrol 1996; 7:2264–2267.

39. Marr KA, Sexton DJ, Conlon PJ, et al. Catheter-related bacteremia and outcome of attempted catheter salvage in patients undergoing hemodialysis. Ann Intern Med 1997; 127:275–280.

40. Sherertz RJ, Ely EW, Westbrook DM, et al. Education of physicians-in-training can decrease risk for vascular catheter infection. Ann Intern Med 2000; 132:641–648.

41. Richet H, Hubert B, Mitemberg G, et al. Prospective multicenter study of vascular-catheter-related complications and risk factors for positive central-catheter cultures in intensive care unit patients. J Clin Microbiol 1990; 28:2520–2525.

42. Charalambous C, Swoboda SM, Dick J, et al. Risk factors and clinical impact of central line infections in the surgical intensive care unit. Arch Surg 1998; 133:1241–1246.

43. Raad II, Hohn DC, Gilbreath BJ, et al. Prevention of central venous catheter-related infections by using maximal sterile barrier precautions during insertion. Infect Control Hosp Epidemiol 1994; 15:231–238.

44. Mimoz O, Pieroni L, Lawrence C, et al. Prospective, randomized trial of two antiseptic solutions for prevention of central venous or arterial catheter colonization and infection in intensive care unit patients. Crit Care Med 1996; 24:1818–1823.

45. Hoffmann KK, Weber DJ, Samsa GP, et al. Transparent polyurethane film as an intravenous catheter dressing: a meta-analysis of the infection risks. JAMA 1992; 267:2071–2076.

46. O'Grady NP, Alexander M, Dellinger EP, et al. Guidelines for the prevention of intravascular catheter-related infections. Infect Control Hosp Epidemiol 2002; 23:759–769.

47. Mermel LA. Prevention of intravascular catheter-related infections. Ann Intern Med 2000; 132:391–402.

48. Veenstra DL, Saint S, Saha S, et al. Efficacy of antiseptic-impregnated central venous catheters in preventing catheter-related bloodstream infection: a meta-analysis. JAMA 1999; 281:261–267.

49. Maki DG, Stolz SM, Wheeler S, et al. Prevention of central venous catheter-related bloodstream infection by use of an antiseptic impregnated catheter: a randomized controlled trial. Ann Intern Med 1997; 127:257–266.

50. Carratala J, Niubo J, Fernandez-Sevilla A, et al. Randomized, double-blind trial of an antibiotic-lock technique for prevention of gram-positive central venous catheter-related infections in neutropenic patients with cancer. Antimicrob Agents Chemother 1999; 43:2200–2204.

51. Schwartz C, Hendrickson KJ, Roghmann K, et al. Prevention of bacteremia attributed to luminal colonization of tunneled central venous catheters with vancomycin-susceptible organisms. J Clin Oncol 1990; 8:1591–1597.

52. Eyer S, Brummitt C, Crossley K, et al. Catheter-related sepsis: prospective randomized study of three methods of long-term catheter maintenance. Crit Care Med 1990; 18:1073–1079.

53. Uldall PR, Merchant N, Woods F, et al. Changing subclavian hemodialysis cannulas to reduce infection. Lancet 1981; 1:1373.

54. Cook D, Randolph A, Sawyer RG, et al. Central venous catheter replacement strategies: a systematic review of the literature. Crit Care Med 1997; 25:1417–1424.

55. Gilbert DN, Moellering RC, Eliopoulos GM, Sande MA, eds. 36th Edition Sanford Guide. Antimicrobial Therapy Inc. 2006:56.

MRSA Bacteremia

Melissa Brunsvold and Lena M. Napolitano
Department of Surgery, University of Michigan Medical System,
Ann Arbor, Michigan, U.S.A.

NOSOCOMIAL BACTEREMIA AND MRSA

Bacteremia is the third most common nosocomial infection, with urinary tract infection most common, and pneumonia ranking second (1,2). The most common causative pathogens for bacteremia are gram-positive pathogens, accounting for 65% of cases, including coagulase-negative staphylococci and *Staphylococcus aureus* (Table 1). The SCOPE project examined 24,179 cases of nosocomial bacteremia in 49 U.S. hospitals between 1995 and 2002, and documented a 10% increase in bacteremia due to gram-positive cocci, with a concomitant 10% decrease in the percentage of bacteremia due to gram-negative bacilli (from 33.2% in 1986 to 23.8% in 2003) (3). *S. aureus* was the second most common bacteremia isolate after coagulase-negative staphylococci, accounting for 20% of cases. Most importantly, the proportion of *S. aureus* bacteremia isolates with methicillin resistance (MRSA) increased from 22% in 1995 to 57% in 2001 (4). In intensive care unit (ICU) patients, 59.5% of all *S. aureus* isolates associated with nosocomial infections are now methicillin-resistant (5). Overall rates of *S. aureus* bacteremia are on the rise; this is due to a significant increase in the rates of MRSA bacteremia.

Initial MRSA clinical isolates were reported in the United States as early as the 1960s, shortly after the introduction of methicillin in 1959 (6). Resistance to methicillin is defined as an oxacillin minimum inhibitory concentration (MIC) of ≥ 4 μg/mL. Isolates that are methicillin resistant are resistant to all beta-lactams. Antibiotic resistance is mediated by the

TABLE 1 Most Common Nosocomial Bacteremia Pathogens in United States

Rank	Pathogen	Percent of all bacteremia isolates	Mortality (%)
1	Coaguloase-negative staphylococci	31.3	20.7
2	*Staphylococcus aureus*	20.2	25.4
3	*Enterococcus* spp.	9.4	33.9
4	*Candida* spp.	9.0	39.2
5	*Escherichia coli*	5.6	22.4
6	*Klebsiella* spp.	4.8	27.6
7	*Pseudomonas aeuruginosa*	4.3	38.7
8	*Enterobacter* spp.	3.9	26.7
9	*Serratia* spp.	1.7	27.4
10	*Acinetobacter baumannii*	1.3	34.0

Source: From Ref. 4.

mec gene on a sequence called the staphylococcal chromosomal cassette (SCC*mec*). There have been five types of SCC*mec* identified. Types I to III are associated with hospital-acquired MRSA and are multi-drug resistant. Type IV is associated with community-associated MRSA and has a more favorable antibiotic susceptibility pattern.

MRSA VS. MSSA BACTEREMIA AND OUTCOMES

Mortality is high in hospitalized patients who develop MRSA bacteremia with reported short-term mortality rates of 12% to 35%. There is general consensus in the published literature that MRSA bacteremia is more likely to be associated with death than methicillin-sensitive *S. aureus* (MSSA) bacteremia (Table 2). A study of 504 bacteremia patients (316 MSSA, 188 MRSA) documented that the overall mortality rate was 22%, but

TABLE 2 Studies Regarding the Effect of Methicillin Resistance and Outcomes in *Staphylococcus aureus* Bacteremia

Ref.	Study design	Total Patient (n)	Patient group	Patients included MRSA	Patients included MSSA	Patient deaths (%) MRSA	Patient deaths (%) MSSA	OR/RR (95% CI)
Whitby et al. (2001) (9)	Meta-analysis of 9 studies	2208	All	778	1430	29	12	2.12 (1.76–2.57) (fixed effect method) 2.03 (1.55–2.65) (random effect method)
Cosgrove et al. (2003) (10)	Meta-analysis of 31 studies	3963	All	1360	2603	Not reported	Not reported	1.93 (1.54–2.42) (random effect model)
Blot et al. (2002) (8)	Cohort study + multivariate survival analysis 2 case-control studies	85	ICU	47	38	53	18	1.93 (1.18–3.18) (hazard ratio)
Talon et al. (2002) (59)	Cohort study, multivariate analysis	99	All	30	69	43.3	20.3	2.97 (1.12–7.88)
Melzer et al. (2003) (60)	Cohort study, logistic regression analysis	815	All	382	433	11.8	5.1	1.72 (0.92–3.20)
Kim et al. (2003) (31)	Cohort study, logistic regression analysis	238	All	127	111	40.2	33.3	In eradicable foci group (n = 96): 0.84 (1.24–2.97) In noneradicable foci group (n = 142): 2.40 (1.19–4.83)
Gastmeier et al. (2006) (11)	National cohort study, multivariable analysis	378	ICU	95	283	16.8	6.0	3.84 (1.51–10.2)

Abbreviations: MRSA, methicillin-resistant *Staphylococcus aureus*; MSSA, methicillin-sensitive *Staphylococcus aureus*; OR, odds ratio; RR, risk ratio.

MRSA bacteremia was associated with a 1.68-fold higher risk of death compared to MSSA patients (7).

MRSA bacteremia in ICU patients was associated with a 1.9-fold increased risk of in-hospital death compared to MSSA bacteremia patients (8). The impact of methicillin resistance on mortality was examined in a meta-analysis of nine studies, concluding that MRSA bacteremia was associated with a two-fold increased risk of death (95% CI, 1.55–2.65) (9). A second meta-analysis of 31 cohort studies (1980–2000, $n = 3963$) determined that MRSA bacteremia was associated with an attributable mortality that was 2.16-fold higher compared to MSSA bacteremia (OR, 1.93) (10). Similarly, a study of 378 cases of *S. aureus* primary bacteremia in ICU patients documented a higher mortality rate in MRSA patients (16.8% vs. 6%) and only MRSA was significantly associated with death from *S. aureus* primary bacteremia (OR, 3.84; CI, 1.51–10.2) (11). Furthermore, community-dwelling, hemodialysis-dependent patients hospitalized with MRSA bacteremia face a higher mortality risk, longer hospital stay, and higher inpatient costs than patients with MSSA bacteremia (12).

MRSA bacteremia is also associated with increased resource utilization. In a study of hospital costs attributable to *S. aureus* bacteremia, it was found that MRSA had nearly twice the cost relative to MSSA ($21,577 vs. $11,668) (13). A study of 348 patients with *S. aureus* bacteremia (96 with MRSA) documented that MRSA bacteremia was associated with significantly increased duration of hospitalization (1.29-fold increase) and hospital charges (1.36-fold increase) (14).

DIAGNOSIS

The diagnosis of MRSA bacteremia is made by isolation of MRSA from blood cultures obtained in patients with presumed systemic infection. Nosocomial bacteremia is defined as a case of bacteremia arising two or more days after admission to hospital as recommended by the Centers for Disease Control (15). Peripheral blood cultures should be utilized for determination of bacteremia whenever possible. The determination of whether the bacteremia is related to an indwelling intravascular catheter is more complex (see Chapter 8). Several methods exist to detect catheter-related bacteremia, and the "paired quantitative blood cultures" method (paired quantitative peripheral and intravascular device blood cultures) is the most accurate method to diagnose catheter-related bacteremia for long-term catheters (16). The national "Guidelines for the Management of Intravascular Catheter-Related Infections" recommend prompt removal of nontunneled central venous catheters and early removal of a tunneled device if there is persistent bacteremia for 72 or more hours of therapy, clinical deterioration, or relapse of bacteremia (17).

RISK FACTORS FOR MRSA BACTEREMIA

A number of risk factors for MRSA bacteremia have been identified including male gender, admission due to trauma, immunosuppression, presence of a central venous catheter or an indwelling urinary catheter, and a past history of MRSA infection (6,18). Other variables associated with MRSA bacteremia include increased age, severe underlying disease (e.g., liver disease, diabetes, renal failure), neurologic disease, intravenous drug use, recent hospitalization, previous antibiotic therapy, and nursing home residence (19,20). Invasive procedures (e.g., catheterization, intubation, surgery) result in disruption of mucocutaneous barriers and are also risk factors. Some experts suggest that the best way to distinguish patients at risk for MRSA is to consider age, underlying medical conditions, previous antibiotic exposure, and the origin of the infection (hospital-acquired, healthcare-associated, or community-acquired). The single most important predictor of MRSA bacteremia is recent prior antibiotic therapy. The presence of decubitus ulcers was also identified as an independent risk factor (21).

Independent risk factors that have been identified for *ICU-acquired* MRSA infections include:

- Hospitalization period in an ICU (OR, 1.090; 95% CI, 1.038–1.144, $P = .001$)

- Central venous catheter insertion (OR, 1.822; 95% CI, 1.095–3.033, $P = .021$)
- Previous antibiotic use (OR, 2.337; 95% CI, 1.326–4.119, $P = .003$)
- Presence of more than two patients having nasal colonization in the same ICU at the same time (OR, 1.398; 95% CI, 1.020–1.917, $P = .037$) (22).

MRSA colonization (either nares or wound) has been confirmed as an independent risk factor for subsequent MRSA infection in ICU patients (OR, 3.84; $P = 0.0003$) (23).

MANAGEMENT OF MRSA BACTEREMIA

Early diagnosis of bacteremia should be sought in order to implement adequate treatment, including prompt appropriate antimicrobial therapy. Inadequate antimicrobial therapy (defined as empiric antibiotic therapy including no antibiotic to which the isolate was susceptible) is a significant risk factor for mortality (24,25). In a study of 549 patients with *S. aureus* sterile site infections, logistic regression analysis identified inappropriate initial antimicrobial treatment as an independent determinant (OR, 1.92) of hospital mortality (26). The importance of *appropriate* (i.e., anti-MRSA) initial empiric antibiotic therapy for patients at risk for MRSA bacteremia is clear. Delay in appropriate antibiotic therapy is also a risk factor for adverse outcome (27). A recent study documented that initial antibiotic therapy was inappropriate in 35% of cases of *S. aureus* bacteremia, and time to effective antibiotic therapy was longer in methicillin-resistant cases (25.5 vs. 9.6 hours; $P < 0.0005$) (28).

S. aureus bacteremia is associated with serious complications including endocarditis in 30% to 40% of cases (29,30). Blood cultures should be repeated three days following initiation of antistaphylococcal antibiotic therapy in all patients with *S. aureus* bacteremia. Patients with positive blood cultures at three days should undergo echocardiography to screen for the presence of endocarditis (Fig. 1). Factors predictive of endocarditis include underlying valvular heart disease, history of prior

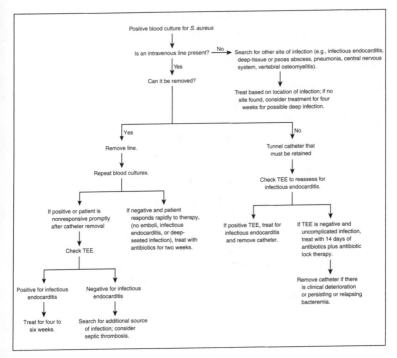

FIGURE 1 Management of *S. aureus* bacteremia. *Abbreviation*: TEE, transesophageal echocardiograpy. *Source*: From: Ref. 58.

endocarditis, intravenous drug use, community acquisition of bacteremia, and an unrecognized source. Hematuria in the setting of staphylococcemia is an important clue to coexisting *S. aureus* infective endocarditis. Hematuria may arise by two mechanisms: renal infarction by embolization or immunologically mediated glomerulonephritis. Transesophageal echocardiography (TEE) can visualize much smaller vegetations and can better detect complications, such as valve perforation and abscesses. Therefore, TEE permits earlier detection and initiation of therapy for endocarditis.

ERADICABLE VS. NONERADICABLE FOCUS OF INFECTION

In addition to antimicrobial therapy, "source control" or "focus identification and eradication" of the MRSA infection is of paramount importance. Drainage of suppurative collections and removal of infected devices that are the source of the MRSA bacteremia are necessary. *Eradicable* foci of MRSA infection include surgically removable infections, drainable abscesses, and indwelling foreign bodies (peripheral and central venous catheters). *Noneradicable* foci of MRSA infection include an unknown primary site, pneumonia, endocarditis, and osteomyelitis or arthritis. Noneradicable focus of infection is an independent predictor of mortality in *S. aureus* bacteremia (31).

A large percentage (25% and higher) of patients with MRSA bacteremia are related to intravascular catheters, which are eradicable foci of infection. Infected intravascular catheters should be promptly removed and placed at a new site, and guidewire exchange of short-term intravascular catheters is contraindicated. Many studies of catheter-associated *S. aureus* bacteremia have documented that prompt catheter removal is associated with a lower risk for endocarditis and greater clinical cure rates.

ANTIBIOTIC TREATMENT OF MRSA AND MSSA BACTEREMIA

Penicillinase-resistant penicillins (methicillin, oxacillin, nafcillin, flucloxacillin) are the antimicrobial agents of choice for *S. aureus* bacteremia due to methicillin-sensitive strains. Vancomycin or first-generation cephalosporins are alternatives but have lower antimicrobial activity than methicillin.

Vancomycin therapy has long been the therapy of choice for MRSA bacteremia. Combination therapy with gentamicin may be useful for the first few days of treatment in selected patients, but there are few prospective randomized data to support the use of combination regimens in *S. aureus* bacteremia. Newer antimicrobial agents, including linezolid, daptomycin, and dalbavancin, also have documented efficacy in the treatment of MRSA bacteremia (Table 3).

Although a rise in community-associated MRSA has been documented in skin and skin-structure infections (32), the vast majority of bloodstream infections are related to healthcare-associated MRSA (33). Other antimicrobial agents that are being used for the treatment of community-associated MRSA skin infections, such as trimethoprim/sulfamethoxazole (TMP/SMX), clindamycin, tetracyclines, and fluoroquinolones, should not be utilized in the treatment of MRSA bacteremia (34).

Vancomycin

Vancomycin has long been the standard treatment for MRSA bacteremia (35). Vancomycin has recently been associated with sub-optimal clinical outcomes. A number of reports have documented persistence of MRSA bacteremia with vancomycin therapy (36,37). Interestingly, vancomycin success in the treatment of MSSA bacteremia may also be problematic in comparison to the semi-synthetic penicillins. Initial vancomycin therapy was also associated with a higher incidence of delayed clearance (≥ 3 days) of MSSA bacteremia (56.3 vs. 37.0%; $P = 0.03$) (24).

Recent studies have identified a relationship between antimicrobial treatment success with vancomycin and decreased vancomycin MICs (≤ 0.5 µg/mL vs. 1.0 to 2.0 µg/mL; $P = 0.02$). Clinical cure rates in bacteremia treatment with vancomycin were higher (55.6%) for patients with MRSA isolates with vancomycin MICs ≤ 0.5 µg/mL whereas vancomycin was only 9.5% effective in cases in which vancomycin MICs for MRSA were higher (1 to 2 µg/mL). A significant risk for vancomycin treatment failure in MRSA bacteremia begins to emerge with increasing vancomycin MICs well within the susceptible range (38). Because of mounting clinical data that suggest a poor response to vancomycin therapy for isolates with a vancomycin MIC of 4 µg/mL, the Clinical

TABLE 3 Antibiotics Available for Treatment of MRSA Bacteremia

Antibiotic	Route	Dose	Advantages	Disadvantages
Vancomycin	IV	1 g IV q12h, titrated by weight and renal function, recommendations to achieve higher trough concentrations (15–20 µg/mL) in pneumonia	Familiarity Low cost	Poor clinical outcome Increased vancomycin MICs Dosage adjustment and monitoring of levels required
Linezolid	IV or PO	600 mg IV q12h	No dosage adjustment in renal or hepatic failure	Thrombocytopenia Cost
Daptomycin	IV	6 mg/kg IV qD	Once-daily dosing	Emerging bacterial resistance Cost
Dalbavancin	IV	1000 mg IV followed by 500 mg IV 1 week later	Once-weekly dosing	Lack of familiarity Cost

Abbreviations: IV, intravenously; MICs, minimum inhibitory concentrations.

and Laboratory Standards Institute has recently lowered the intermediate breakpoint to include vancomycin MICs of 4 μg/mL; MIC breakpoints for vancomycin and staphylococci include the following: susceptible, ≤2 μg/mL; intermediate, 4–16 μg/mL; and resistance, ≥32 μg/mL (39).

In a recent survey of infectious disease consultants asked about persistent bacteremia due to MRSA with a vancomycin MIC approaching the limit of the susceptible range, most indicated that they would switch to newer antimicrobial agents for treatment (40).

Adverse events related to vancomycin include red-man syndrome if the drug is infused too rapidly, and risk for renal toxicity, particularly if utilized with other nephrotoxic drugs such as the aminoglycosides. Increased usage of vancomycin over the past 20 years has also correlated with increased vancomycin-resistant Enterococci (VRE), and VRE colonization is associated with increased risk for VRE infection.

Linezolid

Linezolid is a bacteriostatic oxazolidinone antibiotic that has been proven effective for the treatment of patients with pneumonia and complicated skin and skin-structure infection. Some studies have documented that linezolid has statistically, significantly higher clinical cure rates compared to vancomycin for pneumonia (41) and complicated skin infections (42).

The randomized, open-label, multicenter trial of linezolid versus vancomycin for the treatment of resistant gram-positive infections in children enrolled 113 patients with bacteremia (43). Clinical cure rates were not different for bacteremia patients (84.8% linezolid vs. 80% vancomycin for catheter-related bacteremia; 79.2% linezolid vs. 69.2% vancomycin for bacteremia of unknown source).

A pooled analysis of prospective randomized studies comparing linezolid to vancomycin identified 144 adults with *S. aureus* bacteremia. Of 99 clinically evaluable patients with *S. aureus* bacteremia, primary infection was cured in 55% of linezolid recipients compared to 52% of vancomycin recipients. Clinical cure in MRSA bacteremia patients was

56% for linezolid compared to 46% for vancomycin. No differences in microbiologic success or overall survival were identified between the two groups. In the multivariate analysis, the treatment group was not a significant predictor of clinical cure or survival (44).

A systematic review of the published evidence for linezolid use in treatment of patients with endocarditis suggested that linezolid may be considered as a therapeutic option in the treatment of endocarditis due to multidrug-resistant gram-positive cocci (45). A recently completed prospective study compared linezolid to vancomycin in catheter-related bacteremia, but these data are not yet published.

Adverse events related to linezolid include thrombocytopenia, however the incidence was no different than that related to vancomycin use in the treatment of patients with pneumonia (46).

Daptomycin

Daptomycin is a cyclic lipopetide antibiotic that is rapidly bactericidal in vitro against most clinically relevant gram-positive bacteria, including *S. aureus*. Daptomycin is approved by the FDA for treatment of complicated skin and skin-structure infections at a dose of 4 mg/kg/day IV, and is now approved for the treatment of bacteremia and endocarditis.

An open-label randomized non-inferiority trial compared daptomycin (6 mg/kg IV daily) with standard therapy (vancomycin 1 g IV q 12 hours with appropriate dose adjustment or antistaphylococcal penicillin; with gentamicin 1 mg/kg IV q8 hours for first four days) in patients with *S. aureus* bacteremia with or without endocarditis (47). At the end of therapy, the success rates were 61.7% in the daptomycin group compared with 60.9% in the standard therapy group. Outcome at 42 days after the end of therapy was no different between groups (44.2% daptomycin vs. 41.7% standard therapy, modified intention-to-treat group).

MRSA was isolated from 45 of 120 patients who were treated with daptomycin (37.5%) and 44 of 115 patients who were treated with standard therapy (38.3%). Success rates favored daptomycin over vancomycin among the MRSA cohort (44.4% daptomycin, 31.8% standard therapy, $P = 0.28$) but were higher among patients receiving standard therapy for MSSA infection (44.6% daptomycin, 48.6% standard therapy, $P = 0.74$). This study concluded that daptomycin is not inferior to standard therapy for *S. aureus* bacteremia and right-sided endocarditis.

Importantly, 6 of 19 patients who received daptomycin and had microbiologic treatment failure (32%) were found to have isolates that had developed resistance to daptomycin (MIC ≥ 2 μg/mL). Therefore, if treatment with daptomycin appears to be associated with clinical or microbiologic failure (i.e., persistent fever, symptoms, bacteremia) in patients with bacteremia, the emergence of daptomycin resistance should be carefully assessed. Interestingly, clinically significant renal dysfunction occurred in a significantly lower percentage of patients who received daptomycin compared to standard therapy (11.0% vs. 26.3%, $P = 0.0004$).

Dalbavancin

Dalbavancin is a new, semi-synthetic glycopeptide antibiotic with excellent activity against gram-positive bacteria. Dalbavancin has a long half life (9–12 days), which is longer than that of any currently available glycopeptide. A phase 2, open-label, randomized multicenter study has confirmed the efficacy and safety of weekly dalbavancin therapy for catheter-related bacteremia caused by gram-positive pathogens (48). This prospective trial compared dalbavancin given in two doses administered one week apart, compared with a 14-day course of twice-daily vancomycin in the treatment of adult patients ($n = 75$) with catheter-related bacteremia. The overall success rate for the primary efficacy population (micro-intention-to-treat group = patients infected with a protocol-defined gram-positive pathogen at baseline who received ≥ 1 dose of study medication) for patients treated with dalbavancin was 87% compared with 50% for the vancomycin group. Dalbavancin was statistically superior to vancomycin therapy. Furthermore, both treatment arms were more successful if the catheter was removed than if it was retained at baseline. Dalbavancin is approved by the FDA for treatment of complicated skin and skin-structure infections.

COMPLICATIONS RELATED TO MRSA BACTEREMIA

MRSA bacteremia may lead to several complications including infective endocarditis, sepsis, or metastatic foci of infection. About 12% of patients with *S. aureus* bacteremia have infective endocarditis (49). Metastatic complications, including distant abscesses related to hematogenous dissemination, have been reported in up to 50% of patients with *S. aureus* bacteremia (50,51).

DURATION OF ANTIMICROBIAL THERAPY

The optimal duration of antibiotic treatment for *S. aureus* bacteremia remains unknown. Duration of antimicrobial therapy is dependent on the severity of infection. Recent consensus recommendations for the treatment of *S. aureus* bacteremia suggest that *uncomplicated bacteremia* (defined as isolation of *S. aureus* from blood cultures without endocarditis and without evidence of hematogenous spread) should be treated with intravenous antibiotics for 14 days. *Complicated bacteremia* (defined as persistent bacteremia >72 hours, spread of infection, or infection involving prosthetic devices unable to be removed) should be treated with intravenous antibiotics from 28 to 42 days, based on clinical response to treatment.

There is, however, a lack of data from prospective randomized clinical trials to guide our management. A prospective observational study in 278 patients with *S. aureus* bacteremia determined that duration of antimicrobial treatment ≥14 days was associated with lower mortality (4% vs. 23%) and logistic regression analysis confirmed both duration of antimicrobial therapy ≥ 14 days and focus of infection removal as independent factors associated with reduced mortality (52). Some studies have suggested that a shorter duration of antibiotic treatment is a possible risk factor for recurrence. A retrospective cohort study of 397 patients with *S. aureus* infection complicated by bacteremia documented no association between duration of therapy 14 days or less and recurrence. However, being HIV-infected, having diabetes, or having an infection due to MRSA (OR, 2.11) were independent risk factors for recurrence, and these patients require more careful follow-up (53). Patients with endocarditis require four to eight weeks of intravenous antibiotics with or without surgery.

PREVENTION

Prevention of MRSA bacteremia is the ideal strategy. Previous exposure to antibiotics is the strongest risk factor for MRSA bacteremia (54,55). Minimizing unnecessary exposure to antibiotics is therefore strongly recommended as a preventive strategy. All efforts to prevent catheter-related blood stream infections, including minimizing the use of central venous catheters, should be initiated as a preventive strategy since the presence of a central venous catheter is a significant risk factor for the development of *S. aureus* bacteremia (56). The NNIS system data documented that 87% of blood-stream infections were associated with central venous catheters. The national guidelines for the prevention of catheter-related bacteremia review evidence-based strategies to employ (57).

CONCLUSIONS

Nosocomial bacteremia is a life-threatening infection. Coagulase-negative staphylococci and MRSA are the two most common causative pathogens. Initial empiric antimicrobial therapy for nosocomial bacteremia should include anti-MRSA antibiotics and be administered in a timely manner. Concomitant eradication of the source of the infection, including removal of intravascular catheters if necessary, is an important component of effective therapy.

REFERENCES

1. Richards MJ, Edwards JR, Culver DH, Gaynes RP. Nosocomial infections in medical intensive care units in the U.S. National Nosocomial Infections Surveillance System. Crit Care Med 1999; 27(5):887–892.

2. Richards MJ, Edwards JR, Culver DH, Gaynes RP. Nosocomial infections in combined medical-surgical intensive care units in the U.S. Infect Control Hosp Epidemiol 2000; 21(8):510–515.

3. Gaynes R, Edwards JR, National Nosocomial Infections Surveillance System. Overview of nosocomial infections cuased by gram-negative bacilli. Clin Infect Dis 2005; 41(6):848–854.

4. Wisplinghoff H, Bischoff T, Tallent SM, et al. Nosocomial bloodstream infections in US hospitals: analysis of 24,719 cases from a prospective nationwide surveillance study. Clin Infect Dis 2004; 39:309.

5. NNIS System. National Nosocomial Infections Surveillance (NNIS) System report, data summary from January 1992 through June 2004, issued October 2004. Am J Infect Control 2004; 32:470–485.

6. Barrett FF, McGehee RF, Finland M. Methicillin resistant *Staphylococcus aureus* at Boston City Hostpital. N Engl J Med 1968; 279:441–448.

7. Selvey LA, Whitby M, Johnson B. Nosocomial methicillin-resistant *Staphylococcus aureus* bacteremia: is it any worse than nosocomial methicillin-sensitive *Staphylococcus aureus* bacteremia? Infect Control Hosp Epidemiol 2000; 21(10):645–648.

8. Blot SI, Vandewoude KH, Hoste EA, Colardyn FA. Outcome and attributable mortality in critically ill patients with bacteremia involving methicillin-susceptible and methicillin-resistant *Staphylococcus aureus*. Arch Intern Med 2002; 162:2229–2235.

9. Whitby M, McLaws ML, Berry G. Risk of death from methicillin-resistant *Staphylococcus aureus* bacteremia: A meta-analysis. Med J Aust 2001; 175(5):264–267.

10. Cosgrove SE, Sakoulas G, Perencevich EN, Schwaber MJ, Karchmer AW, Carmeli Y. Comparison of mortality associated with methicillin-resistant and methicillin-susceptible *Staphylococcus aureus* bacteremia: a meta-analysis. Clin Infect Dis 2003; 36(1):53–59.

11. Gastmeier P, Sohr D, Geffers C, et al. Mortality risk with nosocomial *Staphylococcus aureus* infections in intensive care units: results from the German Nosocomial Infection Surveillance System (KISS). Infection 2005; 33(2):50–55.

12. Reed SD, Friedman JY, Engemann JJ, et al. Costs and outcomes among hemodialysis-dependent patients with methicillin-resistant or methicillin-susceptible *Staphylococcus aureus* bacteremia. Infect Control Hosp Epidemiol 2005; 26(2):175–183.

13. Lodise TP, McKinnon PS. Clinical and economic impact of methicillin resistance in patients with *Staphylococcus aureus* bacteremia. Diagn Microbiol Infect Dis 2005; 52(2):113–122.

14. Cosgrove SE, Qi Y, Kaye KS, Harbarth S, Karchmer AW, Carmeli Y. The impact of methicillin resistance in *Staphylococcus aureus* bacteremia on patient outcomes: mortality, length of stay, and hospital charges. Infect Control Hosp Epidemiol 2005; 26(2):166–174.

15. Garner JS, Jarvis WR, Emori TG, Horan TC, Hughes JM. CDC definitions for nosocomial infections. Am J Infect Control 1988; 16:128–140.

16. Safdar N, Fine JP, Maki DG. Meta-analysis: methods for diagnosing intravascular device-related bloodstream infection. Ann Intern Med 2005; 142:451–466.

17. Mermel LA, Farr Bm, Sherertz, et al. Infectious Diseases Society of America, American College of Critical Care Medicine, Society for Healthcare Epidemiology of America. Guidelines for the management of intravascular catheter-related infections. Clin Infect Dis 2001; 32(9):1249–1272.

18. Yoshida T, Tsushima K, Tsuchiya A, et al. Risk factors for hospital-acquired bacteremia. Intern Med 2005; 44(11):1157–1162.

19. Lesens O, Hansmann Y, Brannigan E, et al. Healthcare-associated *Staphylococcus aureus* bacteremia and the risk for methicillin resistance: is the CDC definition for community-acquired bacteremia still appropriate? Infect Control Hosp Epidemiol 2005; 26:204–209.

20. Rezende NA, Blumberg HM, Metzger BS, et al. Risk factors for methicillin-resistance among patients with *Staphylococcus aureus* bacteremia at the time of hospital admission. Am J Med Sci 2002; 323(3):117–123.

21. Lodise TP Jr, McKinnon PS, Rybak M. Prediction model to identify patients with *Staphylococcus aureus* bacteremia at risk for methicillin resistance. Infect Control Hosp Epidemiol 2003; 24(9):655–661.

22. Oztoprak N, Cevik MA, Akinci E, et al. Risk factors for ICU-acquired methicillin-resistant *Staphylococcus aureus* infections. Am J Infect Control 2006; 34(1):1–5.

23. Garrouste-Orgeas M, Timsit JF, Kallel H, et al. Colonization with methicillin-resistant *Staphylococcus aureus* in ICU patients: morbidity, mortality, and glycopeptide use. Infect Control Hosp Epidemiol 2001; 22(11):687–692.

24. Guilarde AO, Turchi MD, Martelli CM, Primo MG. *Staphylococcus aureus* bacteremia: Incidence; risk factors and predictors for death in a Brazilian teaching hospital. J Hosp Infect 2006; 63(3):330–336.

25. Ibrahim EH, Sherman G, Ward S, et al. The influence of inadequate antimicrobial treatment of bloodstream infections on patient outcomes in the ICU. Chest 2000; 118(1):146–155.

26. Schramm GE, Johnson JA, Doherty JA, Micek ST, Kollef MH, Methicillin-resistant *Staphylococcus aureus* sterile-site infection: the importance of appropriate initial antimicrobial treatment. Crit Care Med 34(8):2069–2074.

27. Lodise TP, McKinnon PS, Swiderski L, Rybak MJ. Outcomes analysis of delayed antibiotic treatment for hospital-acquired *Staphylococcus aureus* bacteremia. Clin Infect Dis 2003; 36(11):1418–1423.

28. Khatib R, Saeed S, Sharma M, et al. Impact of initial antibiotic choice and delayed appropriate treatment on the outcome of *Staphylococcus aureus* bacteremia. Eur J Clin Microbiol Infect Dis 2006; 25(3):181–185.

29. Chang FY, MacDonald BB, Peacock JE Jr, et al. A prospective multicenter study of *Staphylococcus aureus* bacteremia: incidence of endocarditis, risk factors for mortality, and clinical impact of methicillin resistance. Medicine 2003; 82:322–332.

30. Fowler VG Jr, Olsen MK, Corey GR, et al. Clinical identifiers of complicated *Staphylococcus aureus* bacteremia. Arch Intern Med 2003; 163:2066–2072.

31. Kim SH, Park WB, Lee KD, et al. Outcome of *Staphylococcus aureus* bacteremia in patients with eradicable foci versus noneradicable foci. Clin Infect Dis 2003; 27:794–799.

32. Moran GJ, Krishnadasan A, Gorwitz RJ, et al.; EMERGEncy ID Net Study Group. Methicillin-resistant *S. aureus* infections among patients in the emergency department. N Engl J Med 2006; 355(7):666–674.

33. Naimi TS, LeDell KH, Como-Sabetti K, Borchardt SM, Boxrud DJ, Etienne J, Johnson SK, Vandenesch F, Fridkin S, O'Boyle C, Danila RN, Lynfield R. Comparison of community- and health care-associated methicillin-resistant *Staphylococcus aureus* infection. JAMA 2003; 290(22):2976–2984.

34. Sabol KE, Echevarria KL, Lewis JS. Community-associated methicillin-resistant *Staphylococcus aureus*: new bug, old drugs. Ann Pharmacother 2006; 40:1125–1133.

35. Markowitz N, Quinn EL, Saravolatz LD. Trimethoprim-sulfamethoxazole compared with vancomycin for the treatment of *Staphylococcus aureus* infection. Ann Intern Med 1992; 117(5):390–398.

36. Khatib R, Riederer KM, Held M, Aljundi H. Protracted and recurrent MRSA bacteremia despite defervenscence with vancomycin therapy. Scand J Infec Dis 1995; 27(5):529–532.

37. Fowler VG Jr, Sakoulas G, McIntyre LM, et al. Persistent bacteremia due to methicillin-resistant *Staphylococcus aureus* infection is associated with *agr* dysfunction and low-level in vitro resistance to thrombin induced platelet microbicidal protein. J Infect Dis 2004; 190:1140–1149.

38. Sakoulas G, Moise-Broder PA, Schentag J, et al. Relationship of MIC and bactericidal activity to efficacy of vancomycin for treatment of methicillin-resistant *Staphylococcus aureus* bacteremia. J Clin Microbiol 2004; 42(6):2398–2402.

39. NCCLS. Performance standards for antimicrobial susceptibility testing: 16th informational supplement. NCCLS document M100-S15. Wayne, PA: NCCLS, 2006.

40. Hageman JC, Liedtke LA, Sunenshine RH, et al. and the Infectious Diseases Society of American Emerging Infections Network. Management of persistent bacteremia cause by methicillin-resistant *Staphylococcus aureus*: A survey of infectious diseases consultants. Clin Infect Dis 2006; 43:e42–e45.

41. Kollef MH, Rello J, Cammarata SK, et al. Clinical cure and survival in Gram-positive ventilator-associated pneumonia: retrospective analysis of two double-blind studies comparing linezolid with vancomycin. Intensive Care Med 2004; 30(3):388–394.

42. Weigelt J, Itani K, Stevens D, et al. Linezolid versus vancomycin in treatment of complicated skin and soft tissue infections. Antimicrob Agents Chemother 2005; 49(6):2260–2266.

43. Kaplan SL, Deville JG, Yogev R, et al. and the Linezolid Pediatric Study Group. Linezolid versus vancomycin for treatment of resistant gram-positive infections in children. Pediatr Infect Dis J 2003; 22(8):877–885.

44. Shorr AF, Kunkel MJ, Kollef M. Linezolid versus vancomycin for *Staphylococcus aureus* bacteraemia: pooled analysis of randomized studies. J Antimicrob Chemother 2005; 56(5):923–929.

45. Falagas ME, Manta KG, Ntziora F, Vardakas KZ. Linezolid for the treatment of patients with endocarditis: a systematic review of the published evidence. J Antimicrob Chemother 2006; 58(2):273–280.

46. Nasraway SA, Shorr AF, Kuter DJ, et al. Linezolid does not increase the risk of thrombocytopenia in patients with nosocomial pneumonia: comparative analysis of linezolid and vancomycin use. Clin Infect Dis 2003; 37(12):1609–1616.

47. Fowler VG Jr, Boucher HW, Corey GR, et al. for the *S. aureus* Endocarditis and Bacteremia Study Group. Daptomycin versus standard therapy for bacteremia and endocarditis caused by *Staphylococcus aureus*. N Engl J Med 2006; 355(7):653–665.

48. Raad I, Darouiche R, Vazquez J, et al. Efficacy and safety of weekly dalbavancin therapy for catheter-related bloodstream infection caused by gram-positive pathogens. Clin Infect Dis 2005; 40:374–380.

49. Fowler VG Jr, Olsen MK, Corey GR, et al. Clinical identifiers of complicated *Staphylococcus aureus* bacteremia. Arch Intern Med 2003; 163:2066–2072.

50. Ringberg H, Thoren A, Lilja B. Metastatic complications of *Staphylococcus aureus* septicemia. To seek is to find. Infection 2000; 28(3):132–136.

51. Gottlieb GS, Fowler VG Jr, Kong LK, et al. *Staphylococcus aureus* bacteremia in the surgical patient: a prospective analysis of 73 postoperative patients who developed *Staphylococcus aureus* bacteremia at a tertiary care facility. J Am Coll Surg 2000; 190(1):50–57.

52. Jensen AG, Wachmann CH, Espersen F, et al. Treatment and outcome of *Staphylococcus aureus* bacteremia: a prospective study of 278 cases. Arch Intern Med 2002; 162:25–32.

53. Kreisel K, Boyd K, Langenberg P, Roghmann MC. Risk factors for recurrence in patients with *Staphylococcus aureus* infections complicated by bacteremia. Diagn Microbiol Infect Dis 2006; 55(3):179–184.

54. Naimi TS, LeDell KH, Como-Sabetti K, Borchardt SM, Boxrud DJ, Etienne J, Johnson SK, Vandenesch F, Fridkin S, O'Boyle C, Danila RN, Lynfield R. Comparison of community- and health care-associated methicillin-resistant *Staphylococcus aureus* infection. JAMA 2003; 290(22):2976–2984.

55. Lodise TP, McKinnon PS, Rybak MJ. Infect Control Hosp Epidemiol 2003; 24(9):655–661.

56. Jensen AG, Wachmann CH, Poulsen KB, et al. Risk factors for hospital-acquired *Staphylococcus aureus* bacteremia. Arch Intern Med 1999; 159:1437.

57. O'Grady NP, Alexander M, Dellinger EP, et al. Guidelines for the prevention of intravascular catheter-related infections; Healthcare Infection Control Practices Advisory Committee. Centers for Disease Control and Prevention. Infect Control Hosp Epidemiol 2002; 23(12):759–769.

58. Bamberger DM, Boyd SE. Management of *S. aureus* bacteremia. Amer Family Physician 2005; 72:2474–2481.

59. Talon D, Woronoff-Lemsi MC, Limat S, et al. The impact of resistance to methicillin in *Staphylococcus aureus* bacteremia on mortality. Eur J Intern Med 2002; 13:31–36.

60. Melzer M, Eykyn SJ, Gransden WR, Chinn S. Is methicillin-resistant *Staphylococcus aureus* more virulent than methicillin-susceptible *S. aureus*? A comparative cohort study of British patients with nosocomial infect and bacteremia. Clin Infect Dis 2003; 37:1453–1460.

Antibiotics for MRSA Infections

R. Lawrence Reed

Surgical Intensive Care Unit, Edward Hines, Jr. Veterans Affairs Hospital
and Department of Surgery, Loyola University Medical Center,
Maywood, Illinois, U.S.A.

Methicillin-resistant *Staphylococcus aureus* (MRSA) is a multidrug-resistant organism. Although "methicillin-resistance" actually means β-lactam antibiotic resistance, there are several other antibiotics that are usually ineffective against MRSA, especially healthcare-associated MRSA (HA-MRSA), such as aminoglycosides and fluoroquinolones.

Despite MRSA's resistance to several antimicrobials, there is a growing list of agents that are effective against the organism. Community-acquired MRSA (CA-MRSA) is often sensitive to many traditional antibiotics, including minocycline, doxycycline, trimethoprim/sulfamethoxazole, rifampin, and clindamycin. HA-MRSA may occasionally be sensitive to these agents, but it is often necessary to use other agents for effective therapy. The rising incidence of MRSA infections has produced a market opportunity for the development of new anti-MRSA antibiotics. Currently, there are four Food and Drug Administration (FDA)-approved antibiotics for the treatment of MRSA infections: vancomycin, linezolid, daptomycin, and tigecycline (Table 1). Knowledge of the risks and benefits associated with each of these agents makes the clinician better able to optimize his patient's care.

VANCOMYCIN

Vancomycin was first discovered in 1956 in some soil samples from southeast Asia, where it was produced by an actinomycete, *Streptococcus*

TABLE 1 Antibiotics Having Food and Drug Administration Approval for Use in MRSA Infections

Drug	Approved indications (MRSA infections)	Routes of administration	Dosing	Comments
Vancomycin	Serious or severe infections (endocarditis, septicemia, bone infections, lower respiratory tract infections, skin, and skin structure infections (53)	Intravenous (orally for *C. difficile* enterocolitis)	1 g every 12 hr	Poor tissue penetration; not as effective against MSSA as β-lactam agents.
Linezolid	cSSTI, pneumonia	Intravenous or orally	600 mg twice daily	Oral bioavailability; excellent tissue penetration; evidence of superiority versus vancomycin for MRSA pneumonia (31,32), cSSTI (54), and SSI (34); evidence of overall reduced costs of treatment, shorter hospital

			lengths of stay, fewer IV days (35,36,54). Higher acquisition costs than vancomycin often provokes restrictions to use.
Daptomycin	cSSTI, bacteremia (including right-heart endocarditis)	Intravenous only	For cSSTI: 4 mg/kg daily For bacteremia: 6 mg/kg	Appears to cover MSSA as well as β-lactam agents and MRSA as well as vancomycin. May be associated with increased incidence of myopathy. Is inactivated by pulmonary surfactant, leading to inferior outcomes for treatment of pneumonia.
Tigecycline	cSSTI, complicated intra-abdominal infections	Intravenous only	100 mg initially, then 50 mg every 12 hr	Very broad spectrum of action. Very high (25–30%) incidence of nausea and vomiting.

Abbreviations: C. difficile, Clostridium difficile; cSSTI, complicated skin and soft-tissue infection; MRSA, methicillin-resistant Staphylococcus aureus; MSSA, methicillin-sensitive Staphylococcus aureus; SSI, surgical-site infections.

orientalis (1). Because of the emergence and prevalence of a penicillin-resistant *S. aureus*, approval of the drug was fast-tracked by the FDA. It was first used clinically in 1958, a mere two years after it had been discovered (1). Early vancomycin preparations were problematic with significant toxicity. Shortly after vancomycin's introduction, however, staphylococcal-resistant penicillins (such as methicillin) and the cephalosporins were developed. These were effective against the penicillin-resistant *S. aureus*. Because of these developments and vancomycin's toxicity, vancomycin use was sparse during its first two decades of clinical use. In the 1970s, the emergence of *Clostridium difficile* produced a new indication for vancomycin. Shortly thereafter, the rising incidence of MRSA caused vancomycin use to escalate to alarming levels.

Vancomycin is a glycopeptide antimicrobial. It binds to the C-terminal end of late peptidoglycan precursors, preventing the effective formation of a bacterial cell wall (2). Its actions against bacteria are carried out on the outer surface of the bacterial cell membrane, as it cannot penetrate into the cytoplasm. Thus, vancomycin depends upon the bacterial translocation of the cell wall precursors onto the outer surface of the microbial membrane. Because vancomycin is effective against cell wall synthesis, it is active only against gram-positive organisms. Gram-positive organisms stain as they do because of the presence of the peptidoglycan cell wall. Gram-negative organisms do not have such a cell wall and are thus unaffected by vancomycin.

Vancomycin is indicated for multiple infections due to gram-positive infections. FDA identifies the minimal inhibitory concentration (MIC) of vancomycin for *S. aureus* as $\leq 4\ \mu g/mL$. Vancomycin intermediately sensitive *S. aureus* (VISA) was initially used to define those organisms with an MIC ranging between 8 and 16 $\mu g/mL$. Vancomycin-resistant *S. aureus* (VRSA) is attributed to those organisms with an MIC of $\geq 32\ \mu g/mL$. Although the vast majority of staphylococci still exhibit MICs in the sensitive range, the ability of vancomycin to achieve tissue levels above the MIC is increasingly questioned. Clinical data indicate that many patients infected with strains of vancomycin-sensitive

S. aureus did not do well despite treatment with vancomycin. The ability of standard doses of vancomycin to clear infection has been related to the plasma levels. Hyatt et al. (3) demonstrated that patients with vancomycin concentrations having an area under the inhibitory curve (AUIC) of >125 had a 97% clinical success rate versus 50% for those with an AUIC < 125. Similarly, Moise et al. (4) demonstrated that patients with an AUIC > 345 had a 78% clinical success rate versus that of 24% for an AUIC of < 346. It should be noted that the AUIC in these studies was dependent upon the MIC, as it was defined by the area under the concentration-time curve divided by the MIC. Sakoulas et al. reported on 30 patients with MRSA bacteremia, in whom multivariate analysis revealed clinical success to be highly correlated with reduced vancomycin MICs (OR 35.46, $P = 0.020$). Patients with an MIC of ≤ 0.5 $\mu g/mL$ had a 55.6% clinical success when treated with vancomycin, whereas those with MICs in the 1.0 to 2.0 $\mu g/mL$ range (previously considered sensitive) only had a 9.5% clinical success rate in response to vancomycin therapy (5). Recently, the Clinical Laboratory Standards Institute dropped sensitivity ranges for *S. aureus* to vancomycin to ≤ 2 $\mu g/mL$, $4-8$ $\mu g/mL$, and ≥ 16 $\mu g/mL$ for sensitive, intermediate, and resistant strains, respectively (6).

Vancomycin is administered intravenously for most infections, except in the occasional management of *C. difficile* enterocolitis, in which it is administered orally. Vancomycin is not absorbed from the oral route, although there have been cases of toxic levels being achieved after oral administration in patients who have had severe mucosal damage of the intestinal tract (7–10). Its apparent volume of distribution approximates total body water (11). However, its penetration into body tissues is relatively poor. Cruciani et al. (12) determined that vancomycin frequently failed to maintain concentrations in lung tissue that exceeded the MIC for susceptible staphylococci. Similar studies in cardiac and valvular tissue have demonstrated barely adequate vancomycin levels (13).

Rapid administration of vancomycin produces an abrupt histamine-like reaction commonly called the "red-man syndrome." Administering the agent over a one-hour infusion time significantly reduces the incidence of this problem. Other idiosyncratic reactions can occur, however, including rashes. Although the early vancomycin preparations were quite toxic, the current formulation is much safer. However, data suggest that administration of the combination of vancomycin and aminoglycoside antibiotics is more nephrotoxic (35%) than either agent alone (7%) (14).

Initial resistance to vancomycin was rare, primarily due to the scant use of the drug. With the emergence of MRSA, vancomycin became more heavily used as it was the primary agent employed for MRSA infections. The resulting increased use and overuse of vancomycin has led to the emergence of vancomycin resistance. Vancomycin-resistant enterococcus (VRE) began to emerge in the late 1980s, VISA emerged in the late 1990s, and VRSA began to emerge in the early 2000s. Thus far, it appears that staphylococcal resistance to vancomycin has been acquired by transfer of a *vanA* gene from a VRE isolate rather than de novo mutation within the *S. aureus* species.

Because of its longevity, vancomycin initially became established as the traditional standard of care for the treatment of MRSA infections. Clinical failure rates of >40% in the treatment of pneumonia have been demonstrated using standard dosing (4,15,16); there is increasing evidence of its shortcomings. MRSA bacteremia in vancomycin-treated patients may persist after defervescence and lead to delayed complications (17).

One study that illuminates vancomycin's shortcoming is that conducted by Gonzalez et al., evaluating 32 cases of a MRSA and 54 cases of methicillin-sensitive *S. aureus* (MSSA) as etiologies of bacteremic pneumonia. Ten of 20 patients (50%) with MRSA pneumonia treated with vancomycin died. Of the cases with MSSA, 47% (8/17) treated with vancomycin died while none (0/10) treated with cloxacillin died. Thus, vancomycin did equally poorly against both MRSA and MSSA (18). Given the significantly better outcome with cloxacillin, the only rationale for vancomycin use is the presence of methicillin resistance. However, this study serves to make it increasingly obvious that vancomycin has some serious shortcomings with respect to its effectiveness.

The need to achieve an adequate tissue concentration, coupled with poor tissue penetration, appears to contribute to outcomes that are worse than one would expect from the microbial sensitivity in the petri dish.

Efforts to improve vancomycin effectiveness have included insuring an adequate trough level (>15 μg/mL) in critical cases, although there are no prospective, randomized, controlled clinical trials indicating that vancomycin efficacy is improved with such a practice, nor can we be assured that vancomycin toxicity will be avoided. There have also been attempts to improve vancomycin effectiveness by combining it with rifampin (19) or aminoglycosides, although, again, there are no prospective data to confirm the validity of this practice. Continuous infusions of vancomycin may offer some advantages over intermittent twice-daily dosing, although such regimens are not considered standard at this time. However, in a prospective, randomized, multicenter trial, Wysocki et al. (20) demonstrated that continuous vancomycin infusion was associated with lower administration costs, more rapid achievement of target concentrations, fewer monitoring samples, and reduced dosing variability in comparison to standard intermittent dosing.

LINEZOLID

Linezolid is the first of a new antibiotic class, the oxazolidinones. It was developed in the 1990s as a response to the rising incidence of MRSA and the increased use and emerging resistance to vancomycin. It was approved for clinical use by the FDA in April 2000. Its mechanism of action involves binding selectively to the bacterial 50S ribosomal subunit, where it inhibits the formation of a functional initiation complex. Linezolid is effective against gram-positive pathogens, such as *Enterococcus faecium*, *S. aureus*, *S. agalactiae*, *S. pneumoniae*, and *S. pyogenes*. It has almost no effect on gram-negative bacteria.

Unique among the anti-MRSA antibiotics is the 100% bioavailability of linezolid. An oral dose of 600 mg of linezolid achieves the same plasma concentrations as the intravenously administered drug. In addition, tissue penetration is generally better than that of many other antibiotics, especially vancomycin. Plasma and epithelial lining fluid (ELF) concentrations of linezolid in healthy volunteers exceeded the minimum concentration needed to inhibit 90% of organisms (MIC90) values for enterococci, staphylococci, and streptococci throughout the entire dosing interval (21). Indeed, it appears that linezolid is concentrated in lung tissue (similar to what has been observed for fluoroquinolones), in that ELF concentrations of linezolid exceed plasma concentrations by a mean of 206% ($\pm$26%) (22,23). Linezolid concentrations in skin blister fluid approach 104% of plasma concentrations (24).

Linezolid is indicated for the treatment of nosocomial pneumonia caused by *S. aureus* (methicillin-susceptible and -resistant strains) or *S. pneumoniae* (including multidrug-resistant strains). It is also indicated in the treatment of complicated skin and skin structure infections, including diabetic foot infections, without concomitant osteomyelitis, caused by *S. aureus* (methicillin-susceptible and -resistant strains), *S. pyogenes*, or *S. agalactiae* (25).

Linezolid is generally well-tolerated. However, there are some adverse effects that have received attention. A reversible myelosuppression (including anemia, leukopenia, pancytopenia, and thrombocytopenia) has been reported in patients receiving linezolid, typically in patients taking the drug for prolonged durations. This has prompted the recommendation that weekly monitoring of complete blood counts be performed in patients taking the drug for more than two weeks. Linezolid has the potential for interaction with adrenergic and serotonergic agents, as it is a reversible, nonselective inhibitor of monoamine oxidase. A review of 15 phase 3 and 4 comparator-controlled clinical trials showed no evidence of an increased incidence of signs and symptoms of serotonin syndrome, in patients treated concomitantly with linezolid and a selective serotonin reuptake inhibitor (26). It should not be used with tyramine-containing foods or pseudoephedrine unless no other options exist. Other side effects include rashes, loss of appetite, diarrhea, nausea, constipation, and fever. A few patients have experienced severe allergic reactions, tinnitus, and pseudomembranous colitis. Presumably because of linezolid's effect on bacterial ribosomes and the similarity to mitochondrial ribosomes, linezolid may be toxic to mitochondria, producing lactic acidosis and peripheral neuropathy in some patients (27). Peripheral neuropathy and optic neuropathy are rarely reported complications (28).

Although its clinical history is relatively brief, resistance to linezolid has already been reported, although rare. Because most bacteria have multiple copies of the 23S rRNA of the 50S ribosomal subunit to which linezolid binds, resistance requires multiple mutations of those copies. Resistance to linezolid was initially reported for VRE isolates, but subsequently observed for *S. aureus*, typically following prolonged courses of linezolid (29). The highest linezolid resistance rate reported thus far is 4% for VRE isolates (30). In 2003, *S. aureus* was first identified as being resistant to linezolid.

Linezolid has been proven effective for the treatment of complicated skin and soft tissue infections (including diabetic foot infections) and for the treatment of pneumonia due to susceptible gram-positive organisms (including MRSA). Recent analyses have been conducted by combining the FDA registration studies for the pneumonia indication to determine if the resulting larger number of study patients could demonstrate against any superiority of linezolid compared to vancomycin. These reports demonstrated improved clinical cure rates and even survival rates for patients who received linezolid for the treatment of MRSA pneumonia (both hospital-acquired and ventilator-associated) than for those treated with vancomycin. Indeed, linezolid therapy fell out as an independent predictor of improved cure and survival (31,32). Similar evidence of superiority over vancomycin has been demonstrated for linezolid treatment of MRSA skin and soft tissue infections, including surgical site infections (33,34). Such improved outcomes using linezolid compared to vancomycin should not come as a surprise, given the improved tissue penetration of linezolid that has already been discussed. Other clinical experience with linezolid has demonstrated a marked reduction in the hospital length of stay, for the treatment of skin and soft tissue infection, as well as a reduced number of IV days (33,35–37). These studies have led to analyses indicating a significant healthcare cost savings, despite the higher acquisition cost of linezolid.

DAPTOMYCIN

Daptomycin is a lipopeptide antibiotic active only against gram-positive organisms. It is a naturally occurring compound which is found in the soil saprotroph, *Streptomyces roseosporus.* Daptomycin binds to bacterial cell membranes in a concentration-dependent and calcium-requiring process, causing rapid depolarization. This results in a rapid bacterial cell death without cell lysis.

Daptomycin has proven in vitro activity against enterococci (including glycopeptide-resistant enterococci), staphylococci (including MRSA), streptococci, and corynebacteria. It was approved for use in skin and skin-structure infections caused by gram-positive infections in September 2003. Daptomycin was shown to have equivalent outcomes to comparator agents including vancomycin or a semisynthetic penicillin. Daptomycin also received FDA approval for the treatment of *S. aureus* bacteremia and right-sided *S. aureus* endocarditis in May 2006.

Despite potent bactericidal activity against *S. pneumoniae*, daptomycin (4 mg/kg every 24 hours) failed to achieve statistical noninferiority against the comparator, ceftriaxone (2 gm every 24 hours). Clinical efficacy in the pneumonia trial was 79% for daptomycin and 87% for ceftriaxone (38). The primary explanation for daptomycin's ineffectiveness in treating pneumonia is that daptomycin interacts with pulmonary surfactant, resulting in inhibition of antibacterial activity (39).

Daptomycin is only available using the intravenous route. Its pharmacokinetics indicate a nearly linear elimination rate. The drug is 92% protein bound, providing a half-life of over eight hours. The drug is typically dosed on a once-daily basis at 4 mg/kg for skin and soft tissue infections, whereas the dose is increased to 6 mg/kg once daily for *S. aureus* bacteremia or right-sided endocarditis.

Although nausea and vomiting are the most common adverse events noted with the drug, their incidence has not been any different from that of the comparator drugs. The specific adverse event that has received most attention, however, is the potential for myalgias and muscle enzyme (CPK) elevations, although this has usually occurred in $<3\%$ of treated patients. Nevertheless, physicians are advised to be alert to the potential for myopathy and rhabdomyolysis during daptomycin therapy. The simultaneous use of daptomycin with statins may potentiate the tendency toward myopathy, leading to the manufacturer's recommendation that statins be discontinued while taking daptomycin.

Because of its unique mechanism of action, it was suggested that daptomycin would be less susceptible to the development of bacterial resistance than other agents. However, resistance has been reported for VRE and *S. aureus* (40–42). In some cases, it appears that resistance is coincident with an increased thickening of the staphylococcal bacterial cell wall, similar to that seen with VISA (43). Microbiological evaluation of daptomycin resistance suggests that resistant organisms frequently lose much of their virulence (44).

TIGECYCLINE

Tigecycline is the first clinically available drug in a new class of antibiotics called the glycylcyclines, which are structurally similar to the tetracyclines in that they contain a central four-ring carbocyclic skeleton. Tigecycline has a substitution at the D-9 position, which is believed to confer broad spectrum activity. Tigecycline targets the bacterial ribosome and is a bacteriostatic agent.

Tigecycline has an extremely broad spectrum of activity, affecting aerobes, anaerobes, gram-positive bacteria (including MRSA), and gram-negative bacteria (including those possessing extended-spectrum β-lactamase plasmids). However, it has no activity against *Pseudomonas* or *Proteus*.

Tigecycline has thus far received approval for the treatment of skin and soft tissue infections as well as intra-abdominal infections. The drug is only available for intravenous infusion, given as an initial 100 mg loading dose followed by 50 mg every 12 hours thereafter. Dose adjustments are necessary for patients with liver disease, but no adjustment is necessary for patients with impaired renal excretion.

OTHER ANTIBIOTICS WITH ACTIVITY AGAINST MRSA

Several older antibiotics have variable activity against MRSA, but do not actually carry FDA approval for the treatment of MRSA infections. Many of these drugs can be administered orally and are often very useful in the treatment of CA-MRSA. Trimethoprim/sulfamethoxazole is often very effective against MRSA microbiologically (45), although in clinical studies it does not perform as well as vancomycin against MRSA (46). Long-acting tetracyclines such as minocycline and doxycycline have also demonstrated effectiveness against MRSA (47). Clindamycin is orally available and often effective against MRSA, although it occasionally develops an erythromycin-induced resistance, identified in the microbiology laboratory by the so-called "D-test" (48). Other agents that are occasionally useful in managing MRSA infections include rifampin, macrolides (i.e., clarithromycin), tetracycline, fluoroquinolones (moxifloxacin and levofloxacin), gentamicin, and chloramphenicol.

There are also antibiotics whose FDA approval is in various stages of approval.

Telavancin

Another drug that will be entering the FDA approval stage very soon is telavancin. This is a lipoglycopeptide that has multiple mechanisms of action. It inhibits cell wall production via inhibition of transglycosylase activity and also disrupts the cell membrane. It demonstrates concentration-dependent killing with the membrane effect occurring at higher concentration levels. Telavancin is bactericidal against MRSA in a murine MRSA pneumonia model (49). Mortality and bacterial clearance was greater for telavancin compared to linezolid or vancomycin.

A phase III trial of complicated skin and soft tissue infection compared telavancin to linezolid and vancomycin. Vancomycin was used in 76% of the patients in the control arm. Overall cure was 80% in both treatment groups; 22 telavancin patients had MRSA isolated and the cure rate was 82% compared to 26 patients in the vancomycin or linezolid treatment arm with a clinical cure rate of 69% (50). The safety profile was similar with nausea being the most common complication in each group. Ongoing studies with gram-positive pneumonia patients are continuing.

Dalbavancin

Dalbavancin, a second-generation lipoglycopeptide agent belonging to the same class as vancomycin, is remarkable for an extremely long half-life that will allow for one-weekly intravenous dosing (51). A skin and soft tissue infection study comparing dalbavancin with linezolid showed equivalent results with 90% of patients in both groups having a successful outcome (52).

Ceftobiprole

Ceftobiprole is a cephalosporin that has been engineered to have activity against many gram-positive organisms including MRSA (53–56). Ceftobiprole is a broad spectrum pyrrolidinone cephem, which is β-lactamase stable and has a strong affinity for the penicillin-binding proteins PBP2a and PBP2x (57–59). The importance of this mechanism of action is that the resistance of MRSA to β-lactams is mediated by PBP2a, which functions after the normal PBPs have been inactivated by β lactams (60,61). Ceftobiprole is β-lactamase stable and has a high affinity for PBP2a, forming a stable acyl-enzyme complex at the active site of PBP2a

(62,63). This creates a very stable inhibition of the enzyme and accounts for its efficacy against MRSA strains.

Ceftobiprole is bactericidal (64–67). It has activity against MRSA, vancomycin intermediate sensitive MRSA, and VRSA (68–70). It also has activity against MRSE. Gram-negative activity appears to be similar to cefepime including pseudomonas, although ESBL activity is not present (71). Anaerobic activity is present for common gram-positive isolates from diabetic foot infections (72). Selection of resistance is assessed as low in comparison to linezolid and moxifloxacin (64). Animal studies demonstrate that ceftobiprole is at least as effective when treating MRSA infections as all currently approved MRSA drugs (66).

Safety data from phase I and II trials are encouraging and raise no serious toxicity questions (61). The drug is cleared by the kidneys and is dosed at 500 mg every 12 hours intravenously. No oral formulation is available. Dosing for pseudomonas coverage is recommended at 500 mg every 8 hours. Phase III trials in patients with complicated skin and soft tissue infection revealed a 93% cure rate for cepftobiprole and vancomycin, which was used as the comparator (61). In patients with MRSA infections, the cure rate for ceftobiprole was 92% versus 90% for vancomycin. Further clinical studies are being completed and FDA approval is being sought in 2007–2008.

REFERENCES

1. Anderson R, Higgins HJ, Pettinga C. Symposium: How a drug is born. Cincinnati J Med 1961; 42:49–60.
2. Courvalin P. Vancomycin resistance in gram-positive cocci. Clin Infect Dis 2006; 42(suppl 1):S25–S34.
3. Hyatt JM, McKinnon PS, Zimmer GS, Schentag JJ. The importance of pharmacokinetic/pharmacodynamic surrogate markers to outcome. Focus on antibacterial agents. Clin Pharmacokinet 1995; 28(2):143–160.
4. Moise PA, Forrest A, Bhavnani SM, Birmingham MC, Schentag JJ. Area under the inhibitory curve and a pneumonia scoring system for predicting outcomes of vancomycin therapy for respiratory infections by *Staphylococcus aureus*. Am J Health Syst Pharm 2000; 57(suppl 2):S4–S9.

5. Sakoulas G, Moise-Broder PA, Schentag J, Forrest A, Moellering RC Jr, Eliopoulos GM. Relationship of MIC and bactericidal activity to efficacy of vancomycin for treatment of methicillin-resistant *Staphylococcus aureus* bacteremia. J Clin Microbiol 2004; 42(6):2398–2402.

6. Performance Standards for Antimicrobial Susceptibility Testing. 16th informational supplement. Wayne, PA: Clinical and Laboratory Standards Institute/ NCCLS, 2006. Report No.: M100-S16.

7. Thompson CM Jr, Long SS, Gilligan PH, Prebis JW. Absorption of oral vancomycin-possible associated toxicity. Int J Pediatr Nephrol 1983; 4(1):1–4.

8. Bergeron L, Boucher FD. Possible red-man syndrome associated with systemic absorption of oral vancomycin in a child with normal renal function. Ann Pharmacother 1994; 28(5):581–584.

9. McCullough JM, Dielman DG, Peery D. Oral vancomycin-induced rash: case report and review of the literature. DICP 1991; 25(12):1326–1328.

10. Aradhyula S, Manian FA, Hafidh SA, Bhutto SS, Alpert MA. Significant absorption of oral vancomycin in a patient with *Clostridium difficile* colitis and normal renal function. South Med J 2006; 99(5):518–520.

11. Reed RL 2nd, Wu AH, Miller-Crotchett P, Crotchett J, Fischer RP. Pharmacokinetic monitoring of nephrotoxic antibiotics in surgical intensive care patients. J Trauma 1989; 29(11):1462–1468; discussion 8–70.

12. Cruciani M, Gatti G, Lazzarini L, et al. Penetration of vancomycin into human lung tissue. J Antimicrob Chemother 1996; 38(5):865–869.

13. Daschner FD, Frank U, Kummel A, et al. Pharmacokinetics of vancomycin in serum and tissue of patients undergoing open-heart surgery. J Antimicrob Chemother 1987; 19(3):359–362.

14. Rybak MJ, Abate BJ, Kang SL, Ruffing MJ, Lerner SA, Drusano GL. Prospective evaluation of the effect of an aminoglycoside dosing regimen on rates of observed nephrotoxicity and ototoxicity. Antimicrob Agents Chemother 1999; 43(7):1549–1555.

15. Fagon J, Patrick H, Haas DW, et al. Treatment of gram-positive nosocomial pneumonia. Prospective randomized comparison of quinupristin/dalfopristin versus vancomycin. Nosocomial Pneumonia Group. Am J Respir Crit Care Med 2000; 161(3 Pt 1):753–762.

16. Malangoni MA, Crafton R, Mocek FC. Pneumonia in the surgical intensive care unit: factors determining successful outcome. Am J Surg 1994; 167(2):250–255.

17. Khatib R, Riederer KM, Held M, Aljundi H. Protracted and recurrent methicillin-resistant *Staphylococcus aureus* bacteremia despite defervescence with vancomycin therapy. Scand J Infect Dis 1995; 27(5):529–532.

18. Gonzalez C, Rubio M, Romero-Vivas J, Gonzalez M, Picazo JJ. Bacteremic pneumonia due to *Staphylococcus aureus*: A comparison of disease caused by methicillin-resistant and methicillin-susceptible organisms. Clin Infect Dis 1999; 29(5):1171–1177.

19. Levine DP, Fromm BS, Reddy BR. Slow response to vancomycin or vancomycin plus rifampin in methicillin-resistant *Staphylococcus aureus* endocarditis. Ann Intern Med 1991; 115(9):674–680.

20. Wysocki M, Delatour F, Faurisson F, et al. Continuous versus intermittent infusion of vancomycin in severe Staphylococcal infections: prospective multicenter randomized study. Antimicrob Agents Chemother 2001; 45(9):2460–2467.

21. Conte JE Jr, Golden JA, Kipps J, Zurlinden E. Intrapulmonary pharmacokinetics of linezolid. Antimicrob Agents Chemother 2002; 46(5):1475–1480.

22. Honeybourne D, Tobin C, Jevons G, Andrews J, Wise R. Intrapulmonary penetration of linezolid. J Antimicrob Chemother 2003; 51(6):1431–1434.

23. Honeybourne D, Tobin C, Jevons G, Andrews J, Wise R. Erratum: Intrapulmonary penetration of linezolid. J Antimicrob Chemother 2003; 52:536.

24. Gee T, Ellis R, Marshall G, Andrews J, Ashby J, Wise R. Pharmacokinetics and tissue penetration of linezolid following multiple oral doses. Antimicrob Agents Chemother 2001; 45(6):1843–1846.

25. Zyvox (linezolid) injection, (linezolid) tablets, (linezolid) for oral suspension. Pharmacia & Upjohn Company, Division of Pfizer Inc., 2006. (Accessed 8/13/2006, at http://www.pfizer.com/pfizer/download/uspi_zyvox.pdf.).

26. Mendelson MH, Hartman CS, Wang Y, Jungbluth GL. Evaluation of potential drug interactions of linezolid with selective serotonin reuptake inhibitors (SSRIs) and other antidepressants: analysis of phase 3 and 4 clinical trials [Poster presentation]. Washington, DC, 2005.

27. Soriano A, Miro O, Mensa J. Mitochondrial toxicity associated with linezolid. N Engl J Med 2005; 353(21):2305–2306.

28. Peppard WJ, Weigelt JA. Role of Linezolid in the treatment of complicated skin and soft tissue infections. Expert Rev Anti-infective Ther 2006; 4(3):357–366.

29. Meka VG, Gold HS. Antimicrobial resistance to linezolid. Clin Infect Dis 2004; 39(7):1010–1015.

30. Paterson DL, Harrison LH, Linden PK, Pasculle AW, Muto CA. Susceptibility of vancomycin resistant *Enterococcus faecium* (VRE) to quinupristin/dalfopristin (Q/D), linezolid (LZD), and daptomycin [abstract K-1409]. In: 43rd Interscience Conference on Antimicrobial Agents and Chemotherapy. Chicago: American Society for Microbiology, 2003:386.

31. Wunderink RG, Rello J, Cammarata SK, Croos-Dabrera RV, Kollef MH. Linezolid vs vancomycin: analysis of two double-blind studies of patients with methicillin-resistant *Staphylococcus aureus* nosocomial pneumonia. Chest 2003; 124(5):1789–1797.

32. Kollef MH, Rello J, Cammarata SK, Croos-Dabrera RV, Wunderink RG. Clinical cure and survival in gram-positive ventilator-associated pneumonia: retrospective analysis of two double-blind studies comparing linezolid with vancomycin. Intensive Care Med 2004; 30(3):388–394.

33. Weigelt J, Itani K, Stevens D, Lau W, Dryden M, Knirsch C. Linezolid versus vancomycin in treatment of complicated skin and soft tissue infections. Antimicrob Agents Chemother 2005; 49(6):2260–2266.

34. Weigelt J, Kaafarani HM, Itani KM, Swanson RN. Linezolid eradicates MRSA better than vancomycin from surgical-site infections. Am J Surg 2004; 188(6):760–766.

35. Li JZ, Willke RJ, Rittenhouse BE, Rybak MJ. Effect of linezolid versus vancomycin on length of hospital stay in patients with complicated skin and soft tissue infections caused by known or suspected methicillin-resistant staphylococci: results from a randomized clinical trial. Surg Infect (Larchmt) 2003; 4(1):57–70.

36. Li Z, Willke RJ, Pinto LA, et al. Comparison of length of hospital stay for patients with known or suspected methicillin-resistant staphylococcus species infections treated with linezolid or vancomycin: a randomized, multicenter trial. Pharmacotherapy 2001; 21(3):263–274.

37. Itani KM, Weigelt J, Li JZ, Duttagupta S. Linezolid reduces length of stay and duration of intravenous treatment compared with vancomycin for complicated skin and soft tissue infections due to suspected or proven methicillin-resistant *Staphylococcus aureus* (MRSA). Int J Antimicrob Agents 2005; 26(6):442–448.

38. Cubist Pharmaceuticals Announces Results from First Phase III Cidecin(R) Community-Acquired Pneumonia Trial Comtex, 2002. (Accessed 8/15/2006, at http://www.corporate-it.net/ireye/ir_site.zhtml?ticker=CBST&script=460&layout=6&item_id=247302.)

39. Silverman JA, Mortin LI, Vanpraagh AD, Li T, Alder J. Inhibition of daptomycin by pulmonary surfactant: in vitro modeling and clinical impact. J Infect Dis 2005; 191(12):2149–2152.

40. Munoz-Price LS, Lolans K, Quinn JP. Emergence of resistance to daptomycin during treatment of vancomycin-resistant Enterococcus faecalis infection. Clin Infect Dis 2005; 41(4):565–566.

41. Lewis JS 2nd, Owens A, Cadena J, Sabol K, Patterson JE, Jorgensen JH. Emergence of daptomycin resistance in *Enterococcus faecium* during daptomycin therapy. Antimicrob Agents Chemother 2005; 49(4):1664–1665.

42. Skiest DJ. Treatment failure resulting from resistance of *Staphylococcus aureus* to daptomycin. J Clin Microbiol 2006; 44(2):655–656.

43. Cui L, Tominaga E, Neoh HM, Hiramatsu K. Correlation between reduced daptomycin susceptibility and vancomycin resistance in vancomycin-intermediate *Staphylococcus aureus*. Antimicrob Agents Chemother 2006; 50(3):1079–1082.

44. Silverman JA, Oliver N, Andrew T, Li T. Resistance studies with daptomycin. Antimicrob Agents Chemother 2001; 45(6):1799–1802.

45. Kaka AS, Rueda AM, Shelburne SA 3rd, Hulten K, Hamill RJ, Musher DM. Bactericidal activity of orally available agents against methicillin-resistant *Staphylococcus aureus*. J Antimicrob Chemother 2006; 58(3):680–683.

46. Markowitz N, Quinn EL, Saravolatz LD. Trimethoprim-sulfamethoxazole compared with vancomycin for the treatment of *Staphylococcus aureus* infection. Ann Intern Med 1992; 117(5):390–398.

47. Ruhe JJ, Monson T, Bradsher RW, Menon A. Use of long-acting tetracyclines for methicillin-resistant *Staphylococcus aureus* infections: case series and review of the literature. Clin Infect Dis 2005; 40(10):1429–1434.

48. Lewis JS 2nd, Jorgensen JH. Inducible clindamycin resistance in Staphylococci: should clinicians and microbiologists be concerned? Clin Infect Dis 2005; 40(2):280–285.

49. Reyes N, Skinner R, Kaniga K, et al. Efficacy of telavancin (TD-6424), a rapidly bactericidal lipoglycopeptide with multiple mechanisms of action, in a murine model of pneumonia induced by methicillin-resistant *Staphylococcus aureus*. Antimicrob Agents Chemotherapy 2005; 49:4344–4346.

50. Stryjewski ME, O'Riordan WD, Lau WK, et al. Telavancin versus standard therapy for treatment of complicated skin and soft-tissue infections due to gram-positive bacteria. Clin Inf Des 2005; 40:1601–1607.

51. Lin SW, Carver PL, DePestel DD. Dalbavancin: A new option for the treatment of gram positive infections. Ann Pharmacother 2006: 40(3):449–460.

52. Jauregui LE, Babazadeh S, Seltzer E, et al. Randomized, double-blind comparison of once-weekly dalbavancin versus twice-daily linezolid therapy for the treatment of complicated skin and skin structure infections. Clin Infect Dis 2005; 41(10):1407–1415.

53. Jones ME, Draghi D, Heep M, Flamm RK, Thornberry C, Sahm DF. Ceftobiprole (BAL9141), an investigational cephalosporin with activity against MRSA, demonstrates in-vitro activity against clinical isolates of *Pseudomonas aeruginosa*. 43rd Infectious Diseases Society of America (IDSA) Meeting; October 6-9, 2005 [abstr. 506].

54. Jones RN, Deshpande LM, Mutnick AH, et al. In vitro evaluation of BAL9141, a novel parenteral cephalosporin active against oxacillin-resistant staphylococci. *J Antimicrob Chemother* 2002; 50(6):915–932.

55. Jones RN, Sader HS, Fritsche TR. In vitro susceptibility testing guidelines for ceftobiprole (BAL9141) using CLSI disk diffusion and broth microdilution MIC methods. Presented at the 45th Annual Interscience Conference on Antimicrobial Agents and Chemotherapy Meeting; Washington, D.C.; December 16–19, 2005. [abstr. D-1647-2005].

56. Jones ME. In-vitro profile of a new β-lactam, ceftobiprole, with activity against methicillin-resistant *Staphylococcus aureus*. Clin Microbiol Infec 2007; 13(suppl 2):17–24.

57. Chambers HF. Evaluation of ceftobiprole in a rabbit model of aortic valve endocarditis due to methicillin-resistant and vancomycin-intermediate *Staphylococcus aureus*. Antimicrob Agents Chemother 2005; 49(3):884–888.

58. Chambers HF. Ceftobiprole: in-vivo profile of a bactericidal cephalosporin. Clin Microbiol Infect 2006; 12(suppl 2):17–22.

59. Chambers, HF. Solving staphylococcal resistance to beta-lactams. Trends Microbiol 2003; 11:145–148.

60. Livermore DM, Pearson A. Antibiotic resistance: location, location, location. Clin Microbiol Infec 2007; 13(suppl 2):7–16

61. Livermore DM. Can beta-lactams be re-engineered to beat MRSA? Clin Microbiol Infect 2006; 12(suppl 2):11–16.

62. Noel GJ, Strauss RS, Pypstra R. Successful treatment of complicated skin and skin structure infections (cSSSI) due to staphylococci, including methicillin-resistant *Staphylcoccus aureus* (MRSA), with ceftobiprole. Presented at the 46th Annual Interscience Conference on Antimicrobial Agents and Chemotherapy Meeting; San Francisco, CA; September 27–30, 2006 [poster L-1212].

63. Noel GJ. Clinical profile of ceftobiprole, a novel β-lactam antibiotic. Clin Microbiol Infec 2007; 13(suppl 2):25–29.

64. Appelbaum P, Hoellman D, Jacobs M. MIC determination of the anti-pneumococcal activity of BAL 9141 compared with other agents [abstract/poster]. The 14th European Congress of Clinical Microbiology and Infectious Diseases, Prague, Czech Republic, May 1–4, 2004. *Clin Microbiol Infection* 2004;10(suppl 3):121.

65. Applebaum PC, Smith K. MIC Values of ceftobiprole and comparators towards *Haemophilus influenzae* and *Moraxella catarrhalis* [abstract]. Presented at the 45th Annual Interscience Conference on Antimicrobial Agents and Chemotherapy Meeting; Washington, D.C.; December 16–19, 2005 [abstr. #E-304-2005].

66. Appelbaum PC. Jacobs MR. Recently approved and investigational antibiotics for treatment of severe infections caused by gram-positive bacteria. Current Opinion Microbiol 2005; 8(5):510–517.

67. Appelbaum PC. MRSA-the tip of the iceberg. Clin Microbiol Infect 2006(Apr); 12(suppl 2):3–10.

68. Bogdanovich T, Ednie LM, Shapiro S, et al. Antistaphylococcal activity of ceftobiprole, a new broad-spectrum cephalosporin. Antimicrob Agents Chemother 2005; 49(10):4210–19.

69. Bogdanovich T, Clark C, Ednie L, et al. Activities of ceftobiprole, a novel broad-spectrum cephalosporin, against *Haemophilus influenzae* and *Moraxella catarrhalis*. Antimicrob Agents Chemother 2006; 50(6):2050–2057.

70. Bogdanovich T, Applebaum PC. Staphylococcal single-step resistance selection studies with ceftobiprole and comparators [abstract]. Presented at the 45th Annual Interscience Conference on Antimicrobial Agents and Chemotherapy Meeting; Washington, D.C.; December 16–19, 2005 [abstr. #F-1163-2005].

71. Goldstein EJ, Citron DM, Merriam VC, et al. The in vitro activity of ceftobiprole against aerobic and anaerobic strains isolated from diabetic foot infections. Antimicrob Agents Chemother 2006; 50(11):3959–3962.

72. Goldstein FW. Combating resistance in a challenging, changing environment. Clin Microbiol Infec 2007; 13(suppl 2):2–6.

Reducing the Risk of Nosocomial Dissemination of MRSA: An Infection Control Perspective

Charles E. Edmiston, Jr.
Department of Surgery, Medical College of Wisconsin,
Milwaukee, Wisconsin, U.S.A.

INTRODUCTION

Staphylococcus aureus has been recognized as a major microbial pathogen for well over 100 years, having the capacity to produce a variety of suppurative and toxigenic disease processes (Table 1). Many of these infections are life threatening, especially in hospitalized patients or individuals with selective risk factors such as diabetes. Within the last 40 years, strains of methicillin-resistant *S. aureus* (MRSA) have rapidly spread throughout the healthcare environment such that it is estimated 20% to 60% of *S. aureus* isolates recovered from hospitalized patients express methicillin resistance (1). Furthermore, a recent study conducted by the Centers for Disease Control and Prevention (CDC) reported that the rate of hospitalization due to MRSA in the United States was highly variable with the rate for MRSA hospitalization in patients under the age of 14 to be 13.1 per 1000 patient discharges, whereas the rate for patients >65 years of age was found to be 63.6 per 1000 patient discharges (2). Recent studies have documented that in addition to increased patient morbidity there is a significant economic burden associated with MRSA infections due to increased length of stay (LOS) and higher related healthcare costs (3,4).

While the prevalence of MRSA isolates within the hospital environment has increased significantly over the past 30 years, two

TABLE 1 Infections Associated with *Staphylococcus aureus*

Skin and soft tissue wounds
Postoperative surgical site infections
Pneumonia
Osteomyelitis
Septic arthritis
Bacteremia
Endocarditis
   Urinary tract
Biomedical device-associated infections

distinct strains (USA300 and USA400) have emerged as important pathogens in individuals lacking the traditional MRSA risk factors and are identified as community-associated MRSA (CA-MRSA). The spectrum of disease, which is caused by these organisms, include skin and soft tissue infections (furuncles, carbuncles, and abscesses) and necrotizing pneumonia (5,6). Unlike hospital-acquired strains of MRSA, CA-MRSA isolates are sensitive to trimethoprim-sulfamethoxazole, gentamicin, tetracycline, and clindamycin; however, selected strains may express an inducible resistance to clindamycin (5,7). While the incidence and clinical significance of CA-MRSA is increasing in the healthcare environment, it is important from an epidemiologic, infection control and treatment perspective to consider these two entities independently and therefore CA-MRSA are reviewed in detail in a separate section of this text (see Chapter 4).

EPIDEMIOLOGY AND PATIENT RISK FACTORS ASSOCIATED WITH MRSA

The gram-positive staphylococci are as a group a major source of patient morbidity in both the hospital and community setting. Table 2 reports the predominant microbial pathogens recovered for hospital-associated

TABLE 2 Predominant Bacterial Pathogens Recovered from Hospital-Associated Infections as Reported from the National Nosocomial Infections Surveillance System Database

| Source | Microorganism | Recovery (%) | | |
		Hospital wide	MICU	SICU
Bloodstream	CoNS	28	36	36
	Staphylococcus aureus	16	13	10
	Enterococci	8	16	15
	Candida spp.	8	11	5
	Escherichia coli	6	3	2
	Enterobacter spp.		3	6
Surgical site	*Staphylococcus aureus*	17		20
	Enterococci	13		8
	CoNS	13		17
	Escherichia coli	9		5
	Pseudomonas seruginosa	8		15
	Enterobacter spp.			1
Respiratory tract	*Pseudomonas aeruginosa*	17	21	17
	Staphylococcus aureus	16	20	17
	Enterobacter spp.	10	9	13
	Staphylococcus pneumoniae	6		
	Haemophilus influenzae	6		
	Klebsiella pneumoniae		8	7
Urinary tract	*Escherichia coli*	25	14	15
	Enterococci	16	14	15
	Pseudomonas aeruginosa	12	10	13
	Candida spp.	9	31	16
	Klebsiella pneumoniae	6		6
	Enterobacter spp.		5	5

Abbreviations: CoNS, coagulase negative staphylococci; MICU, medical intensive care unit; SICU, surgical intensive care unit.
Source: Adapted from Refs. 8–10.

bloodstream, surgical site, respiratory and urinary tract infections based on data obtained from the National Nosocomial Infection Surveillance (NNIS) program administered by the CDC (8–10). Overall, hospital discharges with *S. aureus* infection-related diagnoses are relatively common and as noted earlier, a significant number of hospital-acquired infections associated with *S. aureus* are due to methicillin-resistant strains (20–60%) (1). Nationally, in 1999–2000, the largest percentage of *S. aureus*-related hospitalizations occurred in the southern United States, followed by the Midwest, Northeast, and West. However, the MRSA-related discharge diagnoses were significantly higher ($P < 0.05$) in the Northeast, Midwest, and South compared to the Western states (2).

A myriad of risk factors have been linked to the acquisition and transmission of MRSA within the hospital environment; these include prolonged hospitalization or admission to a long-term care facility (LTCF), diabetes, peripheral vascular disease, recent antimicrobial therapy, intensive care unit (ICU) stay, presence of an invasive indwelling device (intravascular or urinary catheter, endotracheal or tracheostomy tube, etc.), and close contact with colonized individuals (11,12). The proportion of MRSA responsible for infection in the critical care patient population has increased from <30% as reported by NNIS in 1989 to 40% in 1997 (9). Furthermore, several reports have indicated that MRSA infections in the ICU are associated with increased LOS and increased resource utilization (13,14). Specifically, MRSA ventilator-associated pneumonia (VAP) has been documented to independently prolong the duration of ICU hospitalization (15). It is interesting to note that in Scandinavia and The Netherlands the prevalence of HA-MRSA has been less than 1% (13–15). It is suggested that this low prevalence rate is due in part to a nationwide effort to identify colonized patients combined with strict adherence to institutional isolation policies for managing these colonized individuals.

The role of colonization as a risk factor for subsequent dissemination and infection in the ICU patient has been a controversial subject. One study reported that 13.5% of the admissions to the ICU were associated with a positive culture for MRSA at the time of admission or during ICU hospitalization. The rate of importation of MRSA into the ICU as determined by active surveillance culture was 28.6 per 1000 patient days, whereas the rate of acquisition once admitted to the ICU was 6.6 per 1000 patient days. Furthermore, 43.8% of these MRSA-positive patients were detected by active surveillance culture (16). Therefore, this study suggests that dissemination of MRSA within the hospital environment is largely an occult process and that importation of MRSA culture-positive (colonized) patients into the ICU is an important step in the horizontal transmission of these organisms among a high-risk patient population. In a separate study, a prospective analysis was performed to investigate risk factors for ICU-acquired MRSA infections involving ICU and neurologic ICU patients. Nasal cultures were also performed within 48 hours of ICU admission and repeated weekly, until colonization was documented or the patient was discharged. A total of 249 patients were followed over a six-month period; 21 MRSA infections (8.4%) were observed during ICU residency (17). Catheter-related bloodstream infections were the most common MRSA-related infection, followed by pneumonia and surgical site infections. It was reported in this study that 59 patients (23%) were positive for MRSA by nasal culture and 12 of these patients (20.3%) developed a subsequent MRSA infection. Using a univariate analysis, duration of ICU residency, intra-abdominal and orthopedic procedures, mechanical ventilation, central venous line insertion, total parenteral nutrition, previous antibiotic usage, nasal MRSA colonization, and the presence of multiple MRSA colonized-patients in the ICU at the same time were found to be independently associated with MRSA infection.

A study from Scotland suggests that new ICU cases of MRSA are strongly associated with staffing deficits (nursing) and failure of basic infection control practices, including environmental hygiene. The environmental hygiene component is intriguing, since MRSA is rarely viewed as an environmental contaminant like vancomycin-resistant enterococci (VRE) or *Clostridium difficile*. A total of 160 environmental sites (sinks, bedrails, curtains, computer keyboards, etc.) were cultured at selected intervals over a 16-week period. A total of 37 (23%) sites were culture-positive for staphylococci, whereas 26 of the positive cultures (70%) were from sites where frequent hand contact occurred (18). The majority of culture-positive samples revealed coagulase-negative staphylococci; however, in one instance, a MRSA isolate recovered from an environmental site was phenotypically similar to a strain recovered independently from two patients. The relationship of nurse understaffing to the quality of patient care has been clearly addressed in other clinical forums. These data cast suspicion on a documented nursing deficit coupled with poor housekeeping practices serving as a catalyst for subsequent MRSA infections within a susceptible (ICU) patient population.

MRSA has become an important cause of postoperative surgical site infections on all surgical services. Few reports have identified specific risk factors associated with MRSA infections in surgical patients. One study suggests that several postoperative factors play a role in the development of a MRSA infection, including discharge to a LTCF, duration of antimicrobial prophylaxis >1 day, and age ≥ 70 years ($P < 0.05$) (19). The LTCF as a risk factor for postoperative infection is likely due to the probable patient exposure to MRSA within the endemic environment of an LTCF (20). The role of prolonged antibiotic prophylaxis as a postoperative risk factor for MRSA infection is likely more subtle.

A recent study in the author's laboratory suggests that microbial contamination of the surgical wound bed in vascular patients is likely a common occurrence and is more problematic during insertion of a bio-medical device (21). MRSA device-related infections are associated with high patient morbidity and poor clinical outcomes. MRSA was the single most common pathogen (51.6%) associated with acute-onset vascular graft infections (22). Mean hospital stay was reported to be longer in MRSA-infected patients compared to a study cohort of vascular patients with postoperative surgical site infections, and these patients were more likely to undergo an amputation (22). MRSA infection in the vascular patient is a significant independent risk factor associated with in-hospital death (23). Segregation of vascular patients based upon active identification of MRSA patients through surveillance cultures or identification of potential risk factors is effective at reducing the rate of MRSA colonization and infection in patients undergoing aortic or lower limb surgery ($P < 0.001$) (24).

In orthopedic patients, MRSA infections in trauma and elective surgical procedures increased three-fold between 1994 and 2001 (25). Preoperative colonization with MRSA is a risk factor for subsequent infection. Screening and decolonization of MRSA is viewed as a potential strategy for reducing the risk of postoperative infection in patients undergoing prosthetic implantation (26). The incidence of MRSA infection in liver transplant patients is 23% with the sources of infection being vascular catheters, surgical wound, abdomen, and lung (27). A mortality rate of 86% was observed for patients with bacteremic pneumonia (27). The increased risk of infection and mortality has been linked to the high rate of nasal colonization in patients undergoing orthotopic liver transplantation (27,28).

Reports from North America, Europe, and Asia have elevated our concern over the transmission of MRSA between animals and humans. While MRSA infections in animals are considered rare, strains with genetic similarity to hospital-based isolates are emerging in the equine and domestic pet population (29–32). Using an active surveillance screen strategy, MRSA was recovered from 120 (5.3%) nasal swabs in horses admitted to the Ontario Veterinary College. Clinical infection with MRSA was present or developed in 14 (11.7%) of the horses. Horses that were colonized at the time of admission were more likely to develop clinical MRSA infection than noncolonized horses (29). The molecular characteristics of selected strains of MRSA recovered from domestic pets have revealed similar phenotypic (antibiogram) and molecular (*mecA* and *erm* genes) characteristics to human strains (30,31). Asian studies suggest that MRSA strains recovered from both cattle and chickens have some genetic similarity to human strains (32). Finally, a study in a U.K. veterinary hospital confirms that a potential zoonotic linkage may be occurring between veterinary and human strains of MRSA. Swabs were obtained from veterinary staff, hospitalized animals, and environmental surfaces, yielding MRSA from 17.9% of staff members, 9% of the animals, and 10% of the cultured environmental surfaces. Pulse-field gel electrophoresis (PFGE) revealed that 56% of the isolates were genetically similar or identical to one of the two predominant clinical strains found in U.K. hospitals. This study documents the acquisition and dissemination of a clinically significant MRSA strain between humans and pets within a veterinary hospital (33). Transmission of bacterial and viral pathogens from animals to man is not a new concept; however, the role of zoonotic transmission of MRSA is novel and one which may likely have potential clinical significance.

LABORATORY DIAGNOSIS AND EARLY DETECTION OF MRSA

MRSA has become a significant clinical pathogen due to three factors: (*i*) an intrinsic pathogenicity mediated by specific (and often unique) virulence factors, (*ii*) high frequency of nosocomial dissemination and acquisition within the healthcare environment, and (*iii*) limited therapeutic options. Designated strains of hospital-acquired MRSA express resistance to the β-lactam antimicrobial agents and are often resistant to erythromycin, tetracycline, and clindamycin. The rapid identification of an MRSA patient may serve to pre-empt widespread nosocomial dissemination or allow the practitioner to direct appropriate therapy when treating a potentially life-threatening infection. The Clinical and Laboratory Standards Institute (CLSI) recommends one of three testing methods for MRSA: the cefoxitin disk test, the latex agglutination test for penicillin-binding protein 2a (PBP2a), or the oxacillin (6 μg/mL) disk test in Mueller Hinton agar supplemented with 4% (w/v) NaCl (34). The testing procedures also call for incubating test isolates at 33° to 35°C for a full 24 hours before reading the results to identify cells expressing heteroresistance. Staphylococcal resistance to either oxacillin or cefoxitin occurs when the organism carries an altered PBP (PBP2a) that is coded by the *mec*A gene. Oxacillin is stable under storage (refrigerated) condition, and cefoxitin actually is an excellent inducer of the *mec*A gene.

The aforementioned tests represent typical screening strategies for detecting MRSA once an isolate has been recovered from a clinical sample. While conventional culture techniques are highly reliable, the time from sample collection, incubation, isolation to verification of methicillin-resistance can take three to five days (35). Rapid diagnostic testing can confirm the presence of MRSA within a few hours and this information can be used to designate isolation status on general hospital or ICU admission, initiate decolonization protocols in patients undergoing elective surgical procedures, or validate the selection of an appropriate perioperative antimicrobial prophylactic agent. As an infection control tool, rapid diagnostic testing would allow faster detection of MRSA, accelerating implementation of an effective interventional strategy to reduce nosocomial acquisition or dissemination within the hospital environment.

Several molecular techniques have been developed to detect MRSA carriage and many of these assays are based on the detection of *S. aureus* specific genes, specifically the *mec*A gene, which encodes methicillin (oxacillin) resistance. However, most of these techniques required isolation of the organism, often involving multiple steps or a delay of up to 18 hours before strain confirmation. A recent real time (<1 hour) nucleic acid-based polymerase chain reaction (PCR) targets MRSA-specific chromosomal sequences in nasal specimens (specificity 98.4%, positive predictive value of 95.3%, and a sensitivity and negative predictive value of 100%), allowing for rapid detection of MRSA carriers (36). An FDA approved, PCR commercially available kit will detect MRSA nasal and groin carriage within three hours with a sensitivity and specificity in the range of 90–92% (37). Molecular techniques facilitating the rapid detection of MRSA colonization would not only enhance our ability to implement appropriate infection control interventions within a timely fashion, but could be beneficial in identifying high-risk patient populations.

INFECTION CONTROL INTERVENTIONAL STRATEGIES

MRSA Carriage

The mean prevalence of nasal carriage of *S. aureus* in the United States has been reported to be 32.4%, suggesting that a third of the U.S. population is colonized with *S. aureus*. The community carriage of MRSA was determined to be <1.0% (38). However, among individuals recently exposed to selected anti-infectives, the prevalence increases to 4.8%. While asymptomatic colonization with MRSA is a risk factor for subsequent MRSA infection, the use of nasal cultures as a screening tool has been viewed as controversial, with limited clinical relevance. A total of 758 patients admitted to five hospitals were screened for MRSA within 48 hours of admission using conventional culture methodology. A total of 3.4% of patients harbored MRSA in their nares, 19% of patients colonized with MRSA at admission and 25% of patients who acquired MRSA during hospitalization developed an infection with MRSA. These results were significant when compared to methicillin-sensitive *S. aureus* (MSSA) colonized or noncolonized patients ($P < 0.01$) (39). It is likely that some MRSA colonized patients while exhibiting no overt symptoms serve as potential reservoirs for dissemination of resistant staphylococci to other high-risk patient populations. In light of the numerous reports in the literature documenting increased risk for infection associated with MRSA colonized patients admitted to the ICU or undergoing elective surgical procedures, the time may be at hand for screening patients for MRSA colonization, if not as a general rule then possibly in those high-risk patients undergoing invasive medical or surgical procedures (12,16,19,20,22,26,27,40,41).

MRSA Patient Isolation

Regardless of the presence or absence of resistant pathogens within the hospital environment, all healthcare personnel must embrace the fundamental practice of "standard precautions" for all patient populations. Standard precautions imply that all healthcare professionals will use appropriate hand hygiene, gloves, mask (eye protection), gowns, or other personal protective equipment when they anticipate exposure to blood or body fluid, secretion, excretion or contact with mucous membranes or nonintact skin. The use of alcohol-based hand rubs is effective at reducing hand contamination and increasing hand hygiene compliance, especially within the ICU (42,43). Compliance to hand hygiene policies reduce the rate of nosocomial infections and transmission of MRSA (44–46). Unfortunately, hand hygiene compliance remains poor in many institutions as documented by a report demonstrating that 85.2% of patient ICU charts were contaminated with pathogenic or potentially pathogenic bacterial isolates. The contaminating organisms included *P. aeruginosa* and *S. aureus*. MRSA was recovered from 6.8% of the outer surface of patient charts in the ICU (47). It was suggested that more emphasis on hand hygiene compliance is required and that inanimate surfaces may serve as an occult reservoir for resistant nosocomial pathogens.

Patients who are identified as having an MRSA infection are placed in "contact isolation." In addition to standard precaution, contact isolation prevents the transmission of nosocomially important microbial populations, such as MRSA, extended-spectrum β-lactamase (ESBL) resistant bacteria, selective gram-negative-resistant bacteria, VRE, and *C. difficile*. Patients in contact isolation are placed in a private room or cohorted with another patient infected with the same microorganism. Healthcare workers who enter the patient's room must wear gown and glove prior to entry, removing these articles and placing them in an appropriate receptacle before leaving the room. In addition, appropriate hand hygiene must be practiced after leaving the room and before examining or entering another patient's room. While it has been suggested that isolation policies result in diminished patient care and physician contact, no convincing evidence exists to imply that patients are harmed by our current isolation policies. Alternatively, the evidence suggests that contact isolation when coupled with appropriate hand hygiene compliance reduces the dissemination of resistant pathogens, such as MRSA, within the healthcare environment (48,49).

Formulary Considerations

The relationship between antibiotic usage and the rate of MRSA acquisition within the hospital environment is well documented. The use of broad-spectrum cephalosporins and fluoroquinolones is associated with both increased rates of colonization and overt infection in susceptible patient populations (50–52). Two case-control studies found a significant relationship between patient exposure to fluoroquinolones and MRSA colonization or infections (51,53). The effective tissue penetration of the fluoroquinolones leads to the eradication of commensal microbial populations, which colonize the skin surfaces, nares, and other mucous membranes, and create a favorable environment for endemic nosocomial populations to repopulate these sites with resistant strains. Attention to antibiotic stewardship is a key consideration in reducing the risk of MRSA within the healthcare environment. It is proposed that the emergence of antimicrobial-resistant bacterial populations in the ICU can be halted through the process of antibiotic cycling, where the antibiotic formulary is rotated on a 6- to 12-month cycle. Unfortunately, our current understanding of the microbial ecology in the gut or on the surface of the skin suggests a highly complex and intrinsically fluid environment in which antimicrobial cycling alone will not reduce the burden of antibacterial resistance (54). While the perfect strategy is yet to emerge, it is evident that a thoughtful and judicious antimicrobial use policy requires a close collegiality between infection control, pharmacy, microbiology, and the clinical staff.

Decolonization

Mupirocin has been used successfully to decolonize healthcare workers who have been implicated in MRSA outbreaks on both the medical and surgical services. Recently, this agent has been used in combination with active surveillance cultures to identify potential patients colonized with MRSA prior to elective surgical procedures (26,55,56). The use of intranasal mupirocin has also been applied successfully to prevent MRSA infection in the ICU (57). It would appear that mupirocin is effective in eradicating nasal carriage and reducing the risk of infection over the short term; however, the longer-term benefits are presently unknown (58). Furthermore, there is sufficient data to suggest that inappropriate use of mupirocin is associated with (rapid) emergence of resistance, which is highly problematic since mupirocin is currently the only effective agent for MRSA decolonization (59–61).

FINAL CONSIDERATIONS

Infections associated with MRSA are problematic since acquisition and dissemination within the hospital environment is often a failure of adherence to sound, fundamental infection control principles. In the case of catheter-related bloodstream infection (CR-BSI), the prevention of CR-BSI is grounded in the basic principles of infection control, judicious hand washing, and aseptic technique. Rigorous attention to aseptic principles results in decreased infection. While newer technological developments in the area of wound care and the use of antiseptic/antibiotic impregnated devices has been suggested to reduce the risk of CR-BSI, there is no substitution for meticulous catheter care (62–64). Furthermore, to minimize the risk of contamination, all line insertions must be performed under maximal barrier precautions, which require using sterile drapes (large), gowns, masks, and gloves. Several prospective studies demonstrate a significant reduction in catheter colonization, and bacteremia can be achieved using a rigorous aseptic protocol (64). While several surface antiseptics will reduce skin contamination at the insertion site, cleansing with chlorhexidine is superior to elemental iodine or an iodophor (64–66). Two percent chlorhexidine gluconate (CHG) w/v and 70% isopropyl alcohol (IPA) skin-prepping agent demonstrated superior efficacy when compared to povidone iodine (67). Two points are worth considering: (*i*) chlorhexidine exhibits an excellent residual activity compared to other compounds and (*ii*) this agent is not neutralized by blood, serum, or blood proteins (68). A significant national effort exists to reduce the risk of central line—associated infections through use of an evidence-based effort, designated as the "central-line bundle," which comprises several key components including the following:

- Hand hygiene
- Maximal barrier precautions upon insertion
- Chlorhexidine skin antisepsis
- Optimal catheter site selection, with subclavian vein as the preferred site for nontunneled catheters
- Daily review of line necessity with prompt removal of unnecessary lines

S. aureus (MSSA and MRSA) stands out as the most common pathogen associated with pneumonia in the hospital environment. MRSA accounts for up to 14.6% of VAP (41). Mortality rates related to pneumonia have been reported to be significantly greater among patients with MRSA infection (69,70). One should not underestimate the role that hands play in cross-contamination as a mechanism for transmission of healthcare-associated pathogens. Cross-contamination can occur during tracheal suctioning and manipulation of ventilator circuitry or endotracheal tubes. Hand washing is essential when caring for patients on ventilator support. Devices associated with respiratory therapy or diagnostic examination need to be clean/sterilized/disinfected properly since they may serve as a vehicle for dissemination of healthcare-associated pathogens to at-risk patients. The pathophysiology of VAP begins with colonization of the airway and tracheal bronchitis (71,72). Attention to oral hygiene is a fundamental component of any effective strategy for reducing the risk of VAP. Finally, patient head position is a simple means for reducing the rate of VAP. A semirecumbent position (30°–45°) is associated with a lower risk for VAP compared to patients in a supine position (71).

S. aureus is the most common surgical site pathogen, and the incidence of MRSA has increased overall within U.S. hospitals from less than 2.5% in the mid-1970s to greater than 50% in 2003 (73,74). The presence of MRSA in the surgical ICU and other units of the hospital have necessitated the adoption of strict isolation guidelines (48–50). The management of the surgical wound while intrinsically straightforward is often highly variable from institution to institution. The use of sterile gloves and aseptic technique is well documented for the prevention of wound sepsis during the immediate postoperative period. The CDC has suggested that sterile gloves should be used for the first 24 hours of incisional care. No specific glove recommendations are offered for the management of postoperative wounds beyond this period. The use of chemically clean versus sterile gloves for managing wounds is a major discussion point primarily because of the issue of cost (75). The impact of this strategy on infection control practices within an institution is debatable and subject to individual interpretation. Sterile technique, however, is indicated when managing wounds in immunosuppressed patients or open surgical wounds involving exposed organ/space sites.

There are several emerging technologies that may impact infection control practices by reducing the potential for bacterial colonization/contamination of the acute surgical wound. This includes dressings that attempt to manipulate wound biology and accelerate normal wound healing. Another strategy has been the incorporation of antimicrobial or antiseptic substances into the matrix of the wound dressing. The incorporation of silver has potential intrinsic value in reducing MRSA contamination within selected surgical wounds (76,77). Finally, over the past 15 years, numerous antiseptic technologies have been applied to selected biomedical devices (central lines, Foley catheters, shunts, etc.), documenting a reduced infection risk for selected high-risk patient populations. This strategy is extended to selected braided and monofilament sutures in which these devices are coated with an antiseptic agent (triclosan) (78). The presence of a safe, antiseptic device within the wound bed has great appeal, especially in those surgical procedures where the risk of wound contamination is high (79). While innovative technology can play an important role in risk reduction, it is only an adjunctive component of a comprehensive strategy based upon the following surgical cornerstones: timely and appropriate antimicrobial prophylaxis, effective skin antisepsis, and exquisite surgical technique.

Globally, MRSA infections are a significant cause of patient morbidity and mortality, which is unfortunate since many of these infections can be prevented through careful and thoughtful adherence to basic infection control practices. In addition, if we are to reduce the incidence of these infections within the healthcare setting, all healthcare professionals must be aware of the epidemiology, pathogenesis, and recognized mechanisms of microbial transmission/acquisition of MRSA and other drug-resistant bacteria. Looming in the not so distant future is the specter of compulsory (national) reporting of healthcare-associated infection rates (80). It will be interesting to note, based upon historical trends, what if any impact the mandatory reporting of healthcare-associated infections on a state and national level will have on the overall incidence of MRSA infection in the future (81).

REFERENCES

1. Zinn CS, Westh H, Rosdahl VT. An international multicenter study of antimicrobial resistance and typing of hospital *Staphylococcus aureus* isolates from 21 laboratories in 19 countries or states. Microb Drug Resist 2004; 10:160–168.
2. Kuehnert MJ, Hill HA, Kupronis BA, et al. Methicillin-resistant *Staphylococcus aureus* hospitalizations, United States. Emerg Infect Dis 2005; 11:868–872.
3. Engemann JJ, Carmeli Y, Cosgrove SE, et al. Adverse clinical and economic outcomes attributable to methicillin resistance among patients with *Staphylococcus aureus* surgical site infection. Clin Infect Dis 2003; 36:592–598.
4. Cosgrove SE, Sakoulas G, Perencevich EN, et al. Comparison of mortality associated with methicillin-resistant and methicillin-susceptible *Staphylococcus aureus* bacteremia: a meta analysis. Clin Infect Dis 2003; 36:53–59.

5. Fridkin SK, Hageman JC, Morrison M, et al. Methicillin-resistant *Staphylococcus aureus* disease in three communities. N Eng J Med 2005; 352: 1436–1444.

6. Francis JS, Doherty MC, Lopatin U, et al. Severe community-onset pneumonia in healthy adults caused by methicillin-resistant *Staphylococcus aureus* carrying the Panton-Valentine leukocidin genes. Clin Infect Dis 2005; 40:100–107.

7. Lewis JS, Jorgensen JH. Inducible clindamycin resistance in staphylococci: should clinicians and microbiologist be concerned? Clin Infect Dis 2005; 40:280–285.

8. Richards MJ, Edwards JR, Culver DH, et al. Nosocomial infections in medical intensive care units in the United States: National Nosocomial Infections Surveillance system. Crit Care Med 1999; 27:887–892.

9. National Nosocomial Infection Surveillance System. National Nosocomial Infection Surveillance (NIS) system report: data summary from January 1990–May 1999, issued June 1999. Am J Infect Control 1999; 27:520–532.

10. Jarvis WR, Martone W. Predominant pathogens in hospital infections. J Antimicrob Chemother 1992; 29(suppl):19–24.

11. Muto CA, Jernigan JA, Ostrowsky BE, et al. SHEA quideline for preventing nosocomial transmission of multidrug-resistant strains of *Staphylococcus aureus* and enterococcus. Infect Control Hosp Epidemiol 2003; 24:362–386.

12. Marshall C, Wesselingh S, McDonald M, et al. Control of endemic MRSA—what is the evidence? A personal view. J Hosp Infect 2004; 56:253–268.

13. Tiemersma EW, Bronzwaer SL, Lyytikainen O, et al. Methicillin-resistant *Staphylococcus aureus* in Europe, 1999–2002. Emerg Infect Dis 2004; 10:1627–1634.

14. Faria NA, Olivera DC, Westh H, et al. Epidemiology of emerging methicillin-resistant *Staphylococcus aureus* (MRSA) in Denmark: a nationwide study in a country with low prevalence of MRSA infection. J Clin Microb 2005; 43:1836–1842.

15. Vrien M, Blok H, Fluit A, et al. Cost associated with a strict policy to eradicate methicillin-resistant *Staphylococcus aureus* in Dutch university medical center: a 10 year survey. Eur J Clin Microb Infect Dis 2002; 21:782–786.

16. Ridenour GA, Wong ES, Call MA, et al. Duration of colonization and methicillin-resistant *Staphylococcus aureus* among patients in the intensive care unit: implications for intervention. Infect Control Hosp Epidemiol 2006; 27:271–278.

17. Oztoprak N, Cevik MA, Korkmaz AF, et al. Risk factors for ICU-acquired methicillin-resistant *Staphylococcus aureus* infections. Am J Infect Control 2006; 34:1–5.

18. Dancer SJ, Coyne M, Speekenbrink A, et al. MRSA acquisition in an intensive care unit. Am J Infect Control 2006; 34:10–17.

19. Manian FA, Meyer L, Setzer J, et al. Surgical site infections associated with methicillin-resistant *Staphyloccus aureus*: do postoperative factors play a role? Clin Infect Dis 2003; 36:863–868.

20. Rezende NA, Blumberg HM, Metzger BS, et al. Risk factors for methicillin-resistance among patients with *Staphylococcus aureus* bacteremia at the time of hospital admission. Am J Med 2002; 323:117–123.

21. Edmiston CE, Seabrook GR, Cambria RA, et al. Molecular epidemiology of microbial contamination in the operating room environment: is there a risk for infections? Surgery 2005; 138:572–588.

22. Taylor MD, Napolitano LM. Methicillin-resistant *Staphylococcus aureus* infections in vascular surgery: increasing prevalence. Surg Infect 2004; 5:180–188.

23. Cowie SE, Ma I, Lee S, et al. Nosocomial MRSA infection in vascular surgery patients; impact on patient outcome. Vasc Endovascular Surg 2005; 39:327–334.

24. Thompson M. An audit demosntrating a reduction in MRSA infection in a specialized vascular unit resulting from a change in infection control protocol. Eur J Vasc Endovasc Surg 2006; 31:609–615.

25. Nixon M, Jackson B, Varghese P, et al. Methicillin-resistant *Staphylococcus aureus* on orthopaedic wards. J Bone Joint Surg 2006; 88B:812–817.

26. Shams WE, Rapp RP. Methicillin-resistant staphylococcal infections: an important consideration for orthopaedic surgeons. Orthopedics 2004; 27:565–568.

27. Singh N, Paterson DL, Chang FY, et al. Methicillin-resistant *Staphylococcus aureus*: the other emerging resistant gram-positive cocci among liver transplant recipients. Clin Infect Dis 2000; 30:322–327.

28. Desai D, Desai N, Nightingale P, et al. Carriage of methicillin-resistant *Staphylococcus aureus* is associated with increased risk of infection after liver transplantation. Liver Transpl 2003; 9:754–759.

29. Weese JS, Rousseau J, Archambault M, et al. Methicillin-resistant *Staphylococcus aureus* in horses at a veterinary teaching hospital: frequency, characterization, and association with clinical disease. J Vet Intern Med 2006; 20:182–186.

30. Strommenger B, Kehrenbery C, Kettlitz C, et al. Molecular characterization of methicillin-resistant *Staphylococcus aureus* and their relationship to human isolates. J Antimicrob Chemother 2006; 57:461–465.

31. Weese JS, Dick H, Willey BM, et al. Suspected transmission of methicillin-resistant *Staphylococcus aureus* between domestic pets and humans in veterinary clinics and in households. Vet Microbiol 2006; 115:148–155.

32. Lee JH. Occurrence of methicillin-resistant *Staphylococcus aureus* strains from cattle and chickens, and analysis of their *mec*A, *mec*R1 and *mec*I genes. Vet Microbiol 2006; 114:155–159.

33. Loeffler A, Boag AK, Sung J, et al. Prevalence of methicillin-resistant *Staphylococcus aureus* among staff and pets in a small animal referral hospital in the UK. J Antimicrob Chemother 2005; 56:692–697.

34. CLSI 2005. Performance standards for antimicrobial susceptibility testing. CLSI approved standard M100-S15. Wayne, PA: Clinical and Laboratory Standards Institute.

35. Bannerman TL. *Staphylococcus, Micrococcus* and other catalase-positive cocci that grow aerobically. In: Murray PR, Baron EJ, Jorgensenm JH, Pfaller MA, Yolken RH, eds. Manual of Clinical Microbiology. 8th ed. Washington, DC: ASM Press, 2003.

36. Huletsky A, Lebel P, Picard FJ, et al. Identification of methicillin-resistance *Staphylococcus aureus* carriage in less than 1 hour during a hopital surveillance prgram. Clin Infect Dis 2005; 49:976–981.

37. Bishop EJ, Grabsch EA, Ballard SA, et al. Concurrent analysis of nose and groin swab specimens by the IDI-MRSA PCR assay is comparable to analysis by individual-specimen PCR and routine culture assays for detection of colonization by methicillin-resistant *Staphylococcus aureus*. J Clin Microbiol 2006; 44:204–2908.

38. Mainous AG, Hueston WJ, Everett CJ, et al. Nasal carriage of *Staphylococcus aureus* and methicillin-resistant *S. aureus* in the United States, 2001–2002. Ann Fam Med 2006; 4:132–137.

39. Davis KA, Stewart JJ, Crouch HK, et al. Methicillin-resistant *Staphylococcus aureus* (MRSA) nares colonization at hospital admission and its effect on subsequent MRSA infection. Clin Infect Dis 2004; 39:776–782.

40. Cosgrove SE, Qi Y, Kaye KS, et al. The impact of methicillin resistance in *Staphylococcus aureus* bacteremia on patient outcomes: mortality, length of stay and hospital charges. Infect Control Hosp Epidemiol 2005; 26:166–174.

41. Shorr AF, Combes A, Kollef MH. Methicillin-resistant *Staphylococcus aureus* prolongs intensive care unit stay in ventilator-associated pneumonia, despite initially appropriate antibiotic therapy. Crit Care Med 2006; 34: 700–706.

42. Maury E, Alzieu M, Baudel JL, et al. Availability of an alcohol solution can improve hand disinfection compliance in the intensive care unit. Am J Respir Crit Care Med 2000; 162:324–327.

43. Vos A, Widmer AP. No time for handwashing? Handwashing versus alcohol rub; can we afford 100% compliance. Infect Control Hosp Epidemiol 1997; 18:205–208.

44. Pittel D, Hugonnet S, Harbarth S, et al. Effectiveness of a hospital-wide program to improve compliance with hand hygiene. Lancet 2000; 356:1307–1312.

45. Larson EL. APIC guidelines for handwashing and hand antisepsis in healthcare setting. Am J Infect Control 1995; 23:251–269.

46. Boyce JM, Pittet D. Guidelines for hand hygiene in healthcare setting. Recommedations of the Healthcare Infection Control Practices Advisory Committee and the HICPAC/SHEA/APIC/IDSA Hand Hygiene Task Force. MMWR 2002; 51/RR16:1–56.

47. Pathotra BR, Saxena AK, Al-Mulhim AD. Contamination of patient files in intensive care units: an indication of strict handwashing after entering case notes. Am J Infect Control 2005; 33:398–401.

48. Coper BS, Stone SP, Kibbler CC, et al. Isolation measures in the hospital management of methicillin-resistant *Staphylococcus aureus* (MRSA): systematic review of the literature. Brit Med J 2004; 329:533–541.

49. Boyce JM, Havill NL, Kohan C, et al. Do infection control measures work for methicillin-resistant *Staphylococcus aureus*? Infect Control Hosp Epidemiol 2004; 25:395–401.

50. Henderson DK. Managing methicillin-resistant staphylococci; a paradigm for preventing nosocomial transmission of resistant organisms. Am J Med 2006; 119:S45–S52.

51. Graffunder EM, Venezia RA. Risk factors associated with nosocomial methicillin-resistant *Staphylococcus aureus* (MRSA) infection including previous antibiotic use. J Antimicrob Chemother 2002; 49:99–105.

52. Weber SG, Gold HS, Hooper DC, et al. Fluoroquinolones and the risk for methicillin-resistant *Staphylococcus aureus* in hospitalized patients. Emerg Infect 2003; 9:141–142.

53. Dziekan G, Hahn A, Thune K, et al. Methicillin-resistant *Staphylococcus aureus* in a teaching hospital: investigation of nosocomial transmission using a matched case-control study. J Hosp Infect 2000; 46:263–270.

54. Bergstrom CT, Lo M, Lipsitch M. Ecological theory suggests that antimicrobial cycling will not reduce antimicrobial resistance in hospitals. Proc Natl Acad Sci USA 2004; 101:13,285–13,290.

55. Mori N, Hitomi S, Nakajima J, et al. Unselective use of intranasal mupirocin ointment for controlling propagation of methicillin-resistant *Staphylococcus aureus* in a thoracic surgery ward. J Infect Chemother 2005; 11:231–233.

56. Fawley WN, Parnel P, Hall J, et al. Surveillance for mupirocin resistance following introduction of routine perioperative prophylaxis with nasal mupirocin. J Hosp Infect 2006; 62:327–332.

57. Muller A, Talon D, Potier A, et al. Use of intranasal mupirocin to prevent methicillin-resistant *Staphylococcus aureus* infection in intensive care units. Crit Care 2005; 9:R246–R250.

58. Laupland KB, Conly JM. Treatment of *Staphylococcus aureus* colonization and prophylaxis for infection with topical intranasal mupirocin: an evidence-based review. Clin Infect Dis 2003; 37:933–938.

59. Hurdle JG, O'Neill AJ, Mody L, et al. In vivo transfer of high level mupirocin resistance from *Staphylococcus epidermidis* to methicillin-resistant *Staphylococcus aureus* associated with failure of mupirocin prophylaxis. J Antimicrob Chemother 2005; 56:1166–1168.

60. Cavdar C, Atay T, Zeybel M, et al. Emergence of resistance in staphylococci after long-term mupirocin application in patient on continuous ambulatory dialysis. Adv Perit Dial 2004; 20:67–70.

61. Schmitz FJ, Fluit AC, Hafner D, et al. Development of resistance to ciprofloxacin, rifampin and mupirocin in methicillin-susceptible and -resistant *Staphylococcus aureus* isolates. Antimicrob Agents Chemother 2000; 44: 3229–3231.

62. Rupp ME, Lisco SJ, Lipsett PA, et al. Effect of a second-generation venous catheter impregnated with chlorhexidine and silver sulfadiazine on central catheter-related infections. Ann Internal Med 2005; 143:570–580.

63. Lubelchek RJ, Weinstein RA. Strategies for preventing catheter-related bloodstream infections: the role of new technologies. Crit Care Med 2006; 34:905–907.

64. O'Grady NP, Alexander M, Dellinger EP, et al. Guidelines for the prevention of intravascular catheter-related infections. MMWR 2002; 51(No.RR-10): 1–36.

65. Widmer AF. Intravenous-related infections. In: Wenzel RP, ed. Prevention and Control of Nosocomial Infections. Philadelphia: Williams & Wilkins, 1997:771–805.

66. Rubinson L, Wu AW, Haponik EF, Diette GB. Why is it that internists do not follow guidelines for preventing intravascular catheter infections? Infect Control Hosp Epidemiol 2005; 26:525–533.

67. Adams D, Quayum M, Worthington T, Lambert P, Elliott T. Evaluation of a 2% chlorhexidine in 70 isopropyl alcohol skin disinfectant. J Hosp Infect 2005; 61:287–290.

68. Chaiyakunapruk N, Veenstra DL, Lipsky BA, Saint S. Chlorhexidine compared with povidone solution for vascular catheter site care: a meta analysis. Ann Intern Med 2002; 136:792–801.

69. Kollef MH, Shorr A, Tabak YP, Gupta V, Liu LZ, Johannes RS. Epidemiology and outcome of healthcare-associated pneumonia: results from a large US database of culture positive pneumonia. Chest 2005; 128:3854–3862.

70. Rello J, Torres A, Ricart M, et al. Ventilator-associated pneumonia by *Staphylococcus aureus*. Am J Respir Crit Care Med 1994; 150:1545–1549.

71. Flanders SA, Collard HR, Saint S. Nosocomial pneumonia: state of the science. Am J Infect Control 2006; 54:84–93.

72. Tablan OC, Anderson LJ, Besser R, Bridges C, Hajjeh R. Guidelines for preventing healthcare-associated pneumonia. MMWR 2004; 53(RR03): 1–36.

73. Gaynes RP. Surveillance of nosocomial infections: a fundamental ingredient for quality. Infect Control Hosp Epidemiol 1997; 18:475–478.

74. National Nosocomial Infection Surveillance System. National Nosocomial Infections Surveillance (NNIS) system report, data summary from January 1992 through June 2004, issues October 2004. Am J Infect Control 2004; 32:470–485.

75. Wise LC, Hoffman J, Grant L, et al. Nursing wound care survey: sterile and nonsterile glove choice. Wound Ost Cont Nurs 1997; 24:144–150.

76. Edward-Jones V. Antimicrobial and barrier effect of silver against methicillin-resistant *Staphylococcus aureus*. J Wound Care 2006; 15:285–290.

77. Strohal R, Schelling M, Takacs M, et al. Nanocrystalline silver dressing as an efficient anti-MRSA barrier: a new solution to an increasing problem. J Hosp Infect 2005; 60:226–230.

78. Edmiston CE, Goheen MP, Krepel C, et al. Bacterial adherence to surgical sutures: is there a role for antibacterial-coated sutures in reducing the risk of surgical site infections? J Am Coll Surgery 2006; 203:481–489.

79. Ford HR, Jones P, Gaines B, Reblock K, Simpkins DL. Intraoperative handing and wound healing: controlled clinical trial comparing coated Vicryl Plus® suture. Surg Infect 2005; 6:313–321.

80. Rosenstein AH. Hospital report cards: intent, impact and illusion. Am J Med Quality 2004; 19:183–192.

81. McKibben L, Fowler I, Horan T, et al. Ensuring rational public reporting systems for healthcare-associated infections: systematic literature review and evaluation recommendations. Am J Infect Control 2006; 34:142–149.

Outcomes and Cost Considerations with MRSA Infections

Peggy S. McKinnon
Department of Pharmacy, Clinical Research and Infectious Diseases, Barnes-Jewish Hospital, St. Louis, Missouri, U.S.A.

Thomas P. Lodise, Jr.
Department of Pharmacy Practice, Albany College of Pharmacy, Albany, New York, U.S.A.

INTRODUCTION

Over the past two decades, rates of antimicrobial resistance have increased rapidly. Of the two million annual nosocomial infections in the United States, more than 50% are caused by drug-resistant strains of bacteria (1,2). Drug resistance has a considerable impact on patient morbidity and mortality, and is a major economic burden for society with yearly expenditures ranging from US $4 to $30 billion (1–3).

One resistant organism of particular concern is methicillin-resistant *Staphylococcus aureus* (MRSA), which is endemic in many hospitals throughout the world (4). The MRSA rates have been steadily climbing in both the intensive care unit (ICU) and non-ICU hospital setting. Among U.S. hospitals, MRSA is the most commonly isolated antibiotic-resistant pathogen, and accounts for more than half of all *S. aureus* isolates in many institutions (5,6); in domestic ICUs, the MRSA rate exceeds 70% (5).

Historically, MRSA infections have occurred primarily among hospitalized patients, or among those with a history of extensive hospitalization and other predisposing risk factors like indwelling catheters, past antimicrobial use, decubitis ulcers, a postoperative surgical wound, or treatment with enteral feedings or dialysis (7–23). There is,

189

however, growing evidence that suggests the epidemiology of MRSA is evolving: the drug-resistant strain is no longer exclusively confined to hospitals or limited to patients with traditional predisposing risk factors (24–26). Increasingly, reports document nascent community-associated MRSA (CA-MRSA) infection among healthy individuals without known risk factors for MRSA. Outbreaks of CA-MRSA have been reported in close-contact settings, such as prisons, child day cares, sports teams, and Native American Indian communities (27–39). The CA-MRSA is now endemic in certain areas and >10% of patients without a history hospitalization in the preceding year that present to the hospital with a *S. aureus* infection are culture-positive for CA-MRSA (24,27,29).

Vancomycin emerged as the drug of choice for MRSA infection against this backdrop of resistance, and has remained active against MRSA at the currently defined minimum inhibitory concentrations (MICs) breakpoints (5). Within the past 10 years, however, multiple reports have described *S. aureus* strains with reduced susceptibility to vancomycin and some question vancomycin's reduced activity against *S. aureus* with MICs at the high end of the susceptible range (MIC of 2 mg/L) (40–42).

Although contemporary mortality rates are much lower than the pre-antibiotic era, there has been a steady rise in *S. aureus* bloodstream infection (BSI) case-fatality rates (4), and the current mortality rate is reported to be 15% to 60% (7,9,10,12–14,16,17,19,20,22,23,43–49). Inspection of these studies shows that the death rate is usually higher among patients with MRSA–BSI than patients with methicillin-sensitive *S. aureus* (MSSA) BSI; these raise questions regarding how to optimize treatment of serious MRSA infections.

Despite the higher crude mortality rates observed with MRSA–BSI, its role in patient survival has been a contentious issue (7,9,10,12–14, 16,17,19,20,22,23,43–48). This is important to appreciate when attempting to describe attributable outcomes such as cost to the resistance trait. Many believe that the association between MRSA and patient outcomes can be explained by factors other than drug resistance. It is well known that certain medical and comorbid conditions predispose patients to MRSA infection (7,9,10,12–14,16,17,19,20,22,23,43–48). These patient factors may independently contribute to adverse clinical outcomes and obviate an assessment of the relationship between methicillin resistance and patient outcome; indeed, this relationship has been studied extensively with varying conclusions (7,9,10,12–14,16,17,19,20,22,23,43–48).

In an effort to determine the association between MRSA and outcome, Cosgrove et al. (12) performed a meta-analysis to compare mortality rates among patients with BSI caused by MRSA and MSSA. Using the MEDLINE database, these authors reviewed studies that reported mortality rates associated with both MRSA– and MSSA–BSIs from January 1980 through December 2000. Thirty-one cohort studies were identified with a total of 3963 SA-BSI patients; of these, the etiology of the BSI was assigned to MSSA for 2603 (65.7%) patients and MRSA for 1360 (34.3%) patients. Although 24 (77.4%) of the studies did not identify a statistically significant association between methicillin susceptibility and death, the pooled analysis revealed a statistically significant increase in mortality among patients with MRSA bacteremia [36.4% vs. 23.4%, respectively, $P < 0.01$, and pooled odds ratio (OR) of 1.93 (95% confidence interval (CI): 1.54–2.42; $P < 0.001$]. Not surprisingly, Cosgrove et al. tried to overcome the inherent heterogeneity among the studies by creating homogenous subgroups of studies, including a cohort of studies that controlled for disease severity, and examined the relationship between MRSA and death in these comparable subgroups. In all of these subgroup analyses, the OR between MRSA and death consistently remained at 1.56 to 2.2 and the association between MRSA and mortality persisted even when adjustments were made for severity of illness. On the basis of their findings, the authors cited type II error as the primary reason for heterogeneity among results of previous studies (12).

Whitby et al. (48) performed a similar meta-analysis, but limited the analysis to nosocomial BSI caused by *S. aureus*. After a comprehensive literature review of all studies published during the period 1978 to 2000, they identified nine studies comprising of 2209 nosocomial *S. aureus* BSI cases. All but one study found a significant relationship between MRSA and death; similar to the Cosgrove study (12), the relative risk of death was significantly higher for patients with BSI due to MRSA (29%) than MSSA (12%) (OR, 2.12; 95% CI, 1.76–2.57; $P < 0.001$] (48). While further, large-scale studies are needed to determine the definitive contribution of methicillin resistance to observed mortality rates due to MRSA–BSI, these meta-analyses support the notion that the mortality difference between MRSA and MSSA is real, even after adjustment for severity of illness and comorbid conditions, and cannot be solely explained by differences in patient factors.

Despite the ongoing debate about the impact of MRSA on mortality, there is no doubt that MRSA treatment is costly, primarily due to the lengthy hospital stay and the professional costs incurred during admission (Table 1) (7,15,19,43,45,47,49–52). This is exemplified in a study conducted by Rubin et al. (47) who reviewed hospital discharge data from the New York City metropolitan area in 1995 and estimated the incidence, death rate, and cost of *S. aureus* infection (47). During the single year of the study, 13,550 discharged patients had *S. aureus* infections and 2780 (20.5%) of these were MRSA. The attributable cost of CA-MRSA was US \$34,000 compared to \$31,500 for a patient with CA-MSSA. For nosocomial infections, the attributable cost of MRSA was US \$31,400 compared to US \$27,700 for MSSA (47).

These findings have been echoed by multiple other investigators who examined the impact of MRSA in the hospital setting (7,15,19,43,45,49–52). In a study of 348 cases of *S. aureus* BSI (96 cases of MRSA) by Cosgrove et al., both the median length of hospitalization and median hospital charges after onset of *S. aureus* BSI were significantly increased in MRSA patients versus MSSA patients (9 vs. 7 days, $P < 0.05$; US \$26,212 vs. US \$19,212, $P = 0.008$) and these differences persisted following correction for baseline variables [1.29-fold increase in length of stay (LOS), $P = 0.016$; and 1.36-fold increase in hospital charges, $P = 0.017$] (45).

TABLE 1 Comparison of Hospital Costs for Methicillin-Resistant and -Sensitive *Staphylococcus aureus*

Study	Population	Endpoint	MRSA (US$)	MSSA (US$)
Abramson et al. (7)	Nosocomial BSI	Median total cost of hospitalization attributable to BSI	27,083	9661
Capitano et al. (43)	Infections in long-term care facility	Median infection cost	2607	1332
Cosgrove et al. (45)	Nosocomial BSI	Median hospital charges after onset of BSI	26,212	19,212
Engemann et al. (51)	Surgical site infections	Median hospital charges attributable to SSI	92,363	52,791
Lodise and McKinnon (49)	Nosocomial BSI	Adjust mean cost after onset of BSI	21,577	11,668
McHugh et al. (19)	Nosocomial BSI	Mean cost per patient-day of hospitalization	5878	2073
		Adjusted mean cost of initial hospitalization	21,251	13,978
Reed et al. (52)	BSI in dialysis patients	Adjusted mean cost 12 weeks after initial hospitalization	25,518	17,354
Rubin et al. (47)	All infections	Attributable mean cost	34,000	31,500
	Nosocomial infections	Attributable mean cost	31,400	27,700
Wakefield et al. (50)	Nosocomial infections	Mean total cost of hospitalization directly attributable to infection	7481	2377

Abbreviations: BSI, bloodstream infection; MRSA, methicillin-resistant *Staphylococcus aureus*; MSSA, methicillin-sensitive *Staphylococcus aureus*; SSI, surgical site infection.

McHugh et al. reported higher costs among MRSA–BSI than MSSA–BSI. In this study, mean cost per patient-day of hospitalization were US \$3805 higher for MRSA–BSI than for MSSA–BSI (US \$5878 vs. US \$2073; $P = 0.003$). When patients were stratified according to severity of illness as measured by the case mix index, a difference of US \$5302 per patient-day was found between the two groups for all patients with a case mix index greater than 2 ($P < 0.001$) (19). These results were comparable to the study by Wakefield et al. (50), which reported a US \$5000 cost difference between MRSA- and MSSA-hospitalized infections. These cost differences are lower than the median attributable total cost difference reported by Abramson. In this case-control study that matched patients for markers of disease severity, the median cost difference between treating a MRSA–BSI and a MSSA–BSI was US \$17,422 per patient (7). Lodise et al. (49) also noted a stark contrast in LOS and hospitalization costs between MRSA and MSSA bacteremic patients. After adjusting for confounding variables, MRSA bacteremia was associated with a 1.5-fold longer LOS (19.1 vs. 14.2 days, $P = 0.005$) and a two-fold increase in adjusted mean hospitalization costs (US \$21,577 vs. US \$11,668, $P = 0.001$). Similarly, in a case-control study of 121 patients infected with MRSA compared with 123 patients infected with MSSA, Graffunder et al. (15) reported that MRSA-infected patients had a 1.5-fold longer post-diagnosis LOS than MSSA-infected patients.

The methicillin resistance problem is not restricted to the acute care setting, it has also been found to significantly affect the costs associated with management of *S. aureus* surgical site infections (SSIs) (51), *S. aureus* BSI infections among community-dwelling hemodialysis-dependent patients (52), and MRSA infections in long-term care facilities (43). In the SSI study by Engemann et al., the median hospital cost was approximately \$40,000 greater for patients with SSI due to MRSA (median, \$92,363; mean, \$118,415) than for patients with SSI due to MSSA (median, \$52,791; mean, \$73,165; $P < 0.001$). Multivariate analyses were performed and after adjusting for duration of surgery, hospital, length of hospitalization before infection, and comorbid conditions, methicillin resistance was found to be associated with a 1.19-fold increase in the median hospital cost ($P = 0.03$) and the mean cost per case attributable to methicillin resistance was $13,901 per case of *S. aureus* SSI (52).

In a prospective study of MRSA in dialysis patients compared to MSSA bacteremic patients, adjusted costs were higher for patients with MRSA–BSI for the initial hospitalization (US $21,251 vs. US $13,978, $P = 0.012$) and 12 weeks after the initial hospitalization (US $25,518 USD vs. US $17,354, $P = 0.015$) (52). Similarly, the median overall cost associated with MRSA infection in a long-term care facility was reported to be 1.95 times greater than that of MSSA infection (43). Although the magnitude of differences varies between investigations, studies have consistently demonstrated higher hospitalization costs and LOS with MRSA when compared to MSSA infections, typically on the magnitude of 1.2- to 2.0-fold increase in morbidity and costs (53). The observed disparities in study results are most likely secondary to differences in study populations and costing structures. Collectively, these studies establish the gravity of MRSA compared to MSSA with respect to speed of clinical response, length of hospital stay, and cost of hospitalization (7,15,19,43,45,47,49–52).

It is important to note that the above morbidity and cost estimates are conservative and do not account for the additional costs incurred by implementing infection control measures. A Canadian study (54) undertook this analysis by including the cost for isolation and management of MRSA-colonized patients (estimated to be CA $1363 per admission) and the hospital's annual screening cost for MRSA was CA $109,813. Assuming a modest MRSA infection rate of 10% to 20%, they determined the cost associated with MRSA in Canadian hospitals to be CA $42 million to CA $59 million annually (54). Obviously, this would be substantially higher if extrapolated to U.S. hospitals where the average MRSA rate is approximately 50% (5).

Because the morbidity and cost statistics for most of these studies were derived from the hospital perspective, it is important to recognize that this is a limited assessment of the impact of resistance (53).

In addition, most of these figures do not account for the cost of managing MRSA infection outside the hospital, which may include the cost of rehabilitation, extended care facilities, or home intravenous (IV) therapy costs (55). As mentioned previously, vancomycin has historically been the drug of choice for MRSA and can only be used intravenously to treat MRSA infection because the oral formulation is not absorbed. While it is beneficial to treat MRSA patients in the outpatient setting from the payer's standpoint, a recent study reported that the cost of drug acquisition, nursing time, supplies for outpatient IV vancomycin therapy, IV line placement, replacement and management costs, and laboratory costs were quite high and substantially more than the average daily reimbursement of approximately US \$300 estimated from four different healthcare payers (55). In addition, these costs do not quantify the indirect costs or patient impact, which may include the emotional toll of having a drug-resistant infection requiring a hospital isolation room, lost time from work for the patient and family due to a prolonged hospitalization and recovery period, and the long-term health consequences of having a MRSA infection (53).

In summary, MRSA clearly adversely affects both morbidity and mortality and results in a significant cost burden. Additionally, MRSA's impact can be seen in both hospitalized patients and outpatients. Given the continuing increase in the spread of MRSA and the evolution of community-associated strains of MRSA, this pathogen is likely to remain a major challenge for clinicians.

FACTORS CONTRIBUTING TO MRSA IMPACT ON CLINICAL AND ECONOMIC OUTCOMES

The casual pathway for MRSA is complex, and the patient's outcome can be attributed to a confluence of factors related to the organism, treatment, and patient (53). While differences in fitness may explain differences in outcomes (56–60), there are several treatment-related factors to provide a plausible explanation for the greater morbidity, mortality, and cost incurred by MRSA infections. These patients are at an increased risk for delayed administration of effective antimicrobial therapy due to the rising prevalence of multi-drug-resistant MRSA infections (6,24). In a study that examined the relationship between the adequacy of antimicrobial treatment for BSI and clinical outcome among patients requiring ICU admission, 32.9% of MRSA patients did not receive antibiotics that were microbiologically active against the MRSA–BSI at the time of organism identification and antibiotic susceptibility reporting (61). An assessment of 398 patients with *S. aureus* BSI revealed that inappropriate empiric therapy was initiated in 141 patients (35.4%) with MRSA bacteremia (62), and in an outcomes study involving 353 patients, 42.9% of MRSA patients did not receive appropriate therapy within 45 hours of *S. aureus* bacteremia compared to only 9.8% of MSSA patients (46).

These high rates of inadequate empirical therapy are alarming because numerous investigators in various practice settings have correlated the risk of a poor outcome to treatment delays (22,46,61–63). For patients with nosocomial *S. aureus* BSI, Lodise et al. (46) noted that patients with a treatment delay exceeding 45 hours were at an almost three-fold higher risk of mortality compared to patients who received adequate antimicrobial therapy within 45 hours; this study is corroborated by several other investigations (22,23). In addition to the increased mortality risk, delayed treatment drives up the hospital stay and cost. The adjusted mean LOS was longer for patients with delayed treatment compared to those treated effectively within 45 hours of onset of BSI (20.2 vs. 14.3 days, $P = 0.05$) (46). In a *S. aureus* BSI case-control study published recently, MRSA was significantly associated with infection-related mortality and 30-day mortality in the univariate analysis, but this relationship did not persist after adjustment for delayed appropriate treatment in the multivariate analyses. Delayed treatment was highly predictive of both infection-related mortality (OR, 2.2; 95% CI, 1.0–4.5; $P = 0.04$) and 30-day mortality (OR, 2.1; 95% CI, 1.0–4.5; $P = 0.04$) in the multivariate analyses (49). These studies underscore the importance of selecting the appropriate antibiotic early in the course of the infection and may partially explain the negative MRSA outcomes.

A recent study that examined the impact of methicillin resistance on patients with *S. aureus* ventilator-associated pneumonia (VAP) reinforces the importance of appropriate empirical therapy to address poor MRSA outcomes (11). In this study, initial antibiotic therapy was appropriate for every patient and MRSA was not a significant predictor of 28-day mortality in the logistic regression analysis. This study further highlights the need for early MRSA detection and treatment delivery to improve MRSA outcomes, and investigators should continue to monitor the role of such improvements in determining patient outcomes.

Beyond the complications caused by treatment delays, differences in antibiotics play a role in patient outcome for MRSA and MSSA. As previously mentioned, vancomycin has historically been the drug of choice for MRSA, and all of the studies above evaluated MRSA outcomes in the "vancomycin era." Despite its sustained in vitro microbiologic inhibitory activity, researchers are beginning to question the continued utility of vancomycin for MRSA infections (60). Within the past 10 years, multiple reports have described MRSA strains with intermediate susceptibility or high-level resistance to vancomycin (40–42,60). There is also a growing concern that vancomycin resistance to *S. aureus* is underappreciated because the Clinical Laboratory Standard's Institute (CLSI) susceptibility breakpoint is too high (MIC of ≤ 2 mg/L) (60,64). Data, albeit limited, suggest that vancomycin has reduced activity against MRSA infections with vancomycin MIC values at the high end of the CLSI susceptible range (60,64). In a post-hoc examination of 30 MRSA bacteremias from multi-center, prospective vancomycin-refractory compassionate use studies, Sakoulas et al. (64) found that clinical success was highly dependent upon the vancomycin MIC within the CLSI susceptibility range. For MRSA isolates with vancomycin MICs ≤ 0.5 mg/L, vancomycin was 55.6% successful in the treatment of bacteremia, whereas vancomycin was only 9.5% effective in cases in which vancomycin MICs for MRSA were 1 to 2 mg/L. The failure of standard MIC testing methods to detect these patients is concerning because limited data suggests that patients with elevations in vancomycin MICs often have a suboptimal clinical response to vancomycin (65,66).

In vitro data indicates that vancomycin is actually inferior to the β-lactams with respect to the rate of bactericidal activity against MSSA (67), and there is also a growing amount of clinical evidence that suggests that the glycopeptides are inferior to β-lactam antibiotics as therapy for serious staphylococcal infections (14,44,68,69). In a large-scale prospective, multi-center observational study of MSSA–BSI that followed patients for six months after completion of therapy to assess rates of recurrence, nafcillin was superior to vancomycin with respect to preventing bacteriologic failure and relapse, and further, vancomycin use was highly predictive of relapse in the multivariate analysis (OR, 6.5; 95% CI, 1.0–52.8; $P = 0.048$) (44). Mortality was also found to be significantly higher among MSSA-infected patients treated with vancomycin than among those treated with cloxacillin (47% vs. none, $P < 0.01$), in a case-control study of patients with bacteremic pneumonia (14). Furthermore, the relationship between vancomycin therapy and mortality (OR, 14; $P < 0.01$) persisted in the multivariate analysis that adjusted for other variables associated with death.

There is also data to suggest that vancomycin is inferior to linezolid for the treatment of nosocomial pneumonia secondary to MRSA (70,71). In a post-hoc analysis of two prospective double-blind studies of patients with hospital-acquired pneumonia (HAP) (72), clinical cure rates were significantly higher in the linezolid group compared to the vancomycin group (59.0% vs. 35.5%, $P < 0.01$), and this effect persisted in the logistic regression analysis (OR, 3.3; 95% CI, 1.3–8.3; $P = 0.01$) (71). In a similar post-hoc analysis limited to patients with VAP, Kollef et al. (70) also noted significant differences in favor of linezolid over vancomycin in both the *S. aureus* VAP group (48.9% vs. 35.2%, $P = 0.06$), and MRSA–VAP group (62.2% vs. 21.2%, $P = 0.001$). The substandard clinical cure rates observed for vancomycin in these studies may be related to its inability to achieve sufficient concentration in the lungs and epithelial lining fluid (ELF) (73,74). In a vancomycin lung penetration study, the lung tissue:serum concentration ratio ranged from 0.24 to 0.41 at 1 and 12 hours, respectively, after a 1 g dose of vancomycin infused over 30 minutes in a lung penetration lung. More concerning was the fact that nearly half of the patients who had samples measured 12 hours post-dose had undetectable levels of vancomycin in lung tissue. In ELF, the vancomycin blood-to-ELF penetration ratio was reported to be 6:1. Further studies, including prospective randomized clinical trials, are needed to better elucidate the definitive reasons for the low clinical cure rates observed for vancomycin among patients with HAP and VAP.

A recent prospective pharmacoeconomic model was conducted to determine the incremental cost-effectiveness of linezolid compared with vancomycin for the treatment of VAP due to *S. aureus* (75). Investigators conducted a decision model analysis of the cost and efficacy of linezolid versus vancomycin. The primary outcome was the incremental cost-effectiveness of linezolid in terms of cost per added quality-adjusted life-year (QALY) gained. Model estimates were derived from prospective trials of linezolid for VAP and from other studies describing the costs and outcomes for VAP. Despite its higher cost, linezolid was cost-effective for the treatment of VAP. The cost per QALY equals approximately $30,000. This is less than the accepted standard of $100,000 per QALY for cost-effectiveness analysis in healthcare. The authors concluded that line-zolid is a cost-effective alternative to vancomycin for the treatment of VAP. Although the acquisition cost of linezolid is significantly more expensive than vancomycin, the efficacy of linezolid compensates for the cost differential. Conclusions were found to be robust across a wide range of values for the model uncertainties (75).

In addition, linezolid has demonstrated higher clinical and microbio-logical success rates for MRSA SSIs and complicated skin and soft tissue infections (cSSTI) (76,77). In an open-label, comparator-controlled, multicenter study that included patients with suspected or proven

MRSA-complicated skin and soft tissue infections, linezolid clinical cure rates were similar to vancomycin at the test of cure (TOC) visit in the intent to treat population, and superior to vancomycin (88.6% and 66.9%, respectively, $P < 0.001$) at the TOC visit for patients with documented MRSA ($P < 0.001$) (76). In another open-label, comparator-controlled study that involved patients with known or suspected MRSA SSIs (77), linezolid produced significantly more microbiologically cured patients compared to vancomycin (87% vs. 48%, respectively; 95% CI, 16.51, 60.27; $P = 0.0022$).

Another demonstrated advantage is that linezolid is available as a 100% bioavailable oral treatment for MRSA infection. Until the availability of linezolid, no proven oral treatment option was available for MRSA patients who are typically treated with intravenous vancomycin and remain hospitalized for the duration of their treatment. This not only places the patients at risk for other nosocomial infections, but also increases the most costly component of infection management: the cost of hospitalization. The availability of antibiotics with highly bioavailable oral formulations enables clinicians to switch their patients to oral dosing, thereby allowing the patient to be discharged earlier. In a recent survey of internal medicine and infectious diseases, doctors indicate that they would be more inclined to discharge MRSA patients earlier if a high-bioavailability oral formulation existed (78).

In order to determine the potential cost saving of an early switch to oral linezolid or early hospital discharge, Parodi et al. (79) conducted a retrospective cohort study at the Veterans Administration Greater Los Angeles Healthcare System. Of the 172 patients who fulfilled the inclusion criteria, 103 (58.2%) were potentially eligible for switching to oral linezolid and 55 (32.0%) were eligible for early discharge. Investigators found that the mean savings per eligible treatment course in vancomycin therapy and LOS were 5.2 and 3.3 days, respectively, and the overall potential savings totaled US \$220,181 with a mean savings per treatment course of US \$4003. Examination of the economic outcomes of patients with known or suspected MRSA infection treated with linezolid or vancomycin in phase III and IV trials has validated this position (76,77,80–84). These studies have consistently demonstrated the economic benefits of linezolid compared to vancomycin due to decreased LOS, duration of IV therapy, and cost of care; when coupled with the human benefit of reduced morbidity and mortality, the evidence for new treatment options against MRSA is compelling. In the aforementioned vancomycin versus linezolid cSSTI study (84), IV duration of therapy was shortened from 12.6 to 1.8 days and hospital LOS was reduced from 10.7 to 8.1 days in MRSA patients with cSSTI-treated with linezolid compared to vancomycin. Furthermore, McKinnon et al. (83) observed a cost difference of $1125 per patient in favor of linezolid ($4881 vs. $6006 for vancomycin-treated patients) when costs of drug, concomitant medications, procedures, and hospital costs were analyzed for the U.S. subset of patients with MRSA–cSSTI (83). Although other newer agents have been studied for MRSA infection, at the present time, the authors are unaware of any improved outcomes or economic benefit described with daptomycin, tigecycline, or quinupristin/dalfopristin for MRSA treatment. Continued evaluation of new agents against MRSA will shed additional light on the potential role of the treatment effect.

CONCLUSIONS

Rates of MRSA in the hospital and the community continue to increase. High patient morbidity, mortality, and resulting healthcare resource utilization are associated with MRSA when compared to MSSA. Studies evaluating the clinical and economic impact of MRSA compared to MSSA have consistently identified divergent patient outcomes. Numerous investigations have attempted to control for factors that may contribute to such systematic differences, yet none have controlled for all variables, including delayed treatment and antibiotic selection. Although the data are not definitive, it appears that treatment-related factors may be primarily responsible for the negative outcomes observed with MRSA, as most studies demonstrating the negative patient outcomes and increase in cost were performed when vancomycin was the mainstay of treatment for MRSA.

The role of vancomycin in the treatment of MRSA infections has recently been questioned, and there is a growing amount of clinical evidence that confirms the suboptimal response of MRSA to vancomycin, particularly for nosocomial pneumonia and skin and soft tissue infections. Undoubtedly, antibiotics with good bioavailability, such as linezolid, have been shown to facilitate early discharge and alleviate the economic burden of hospitalization for MRSA infections. In the era of newer agents, such as linezolid, daptomycin, and tigecycline, we will begin to learn more about the treatment-related factors, specifically antibiotic selection, that impact patient outcomes. Further studies are needed to determine if these new agents will replace vancomycin as the drug of choice for MRSA infection and remedy the adverse clinical and economic outcomes frequently observed with MRSA infections.

REFERENCES

1. Weinstein RA. Nosocomial infection update. Emerg Infect Dis 1998; 4:416–420.
2. Jones RN. Resistance patterns among nosocomial pathogens: trends over the past few years. Chest 2001; 119:397S–404S.
3. Neu HC. The crisis in antibiotic resistance. Science 1992; 257:1064–1073.
4. Panlilio AL, Culver DH, Gaynes RP, et al. Methicillin-resistant *Staphylococcus aureus* in U.S. hospitals, 1975–1991. Infect Control Hosp Epidemiol 1992; 13:582–586.
5. National Nosocomial Infections Surveillance (NNIS) System Report, data summary from January 1992 through June 2004, issued October 2004. Am J Infect Control 2004; 32:470–485.
6. Streit JM, Jones RN, Sader HS, Fritsche TR. Assessment of pathogen occurrences and resistance profiles among infected patients in the intensive care unit: report from the SENTRY Antimicrobial Surveillance Program (North America, 2001). Int J Antimicrob Agents 2004; 24:111–118.

7. Abramson MA, Sexton DJ. Nosocomial methicillin-resistant and methicillin-susceptible *Staphylococcus aureus* primary bacteremia: at what costs? Infect Control Hosp Epidemiol 1999; 20:408–411.

8. Asensio A, Guerrero A, Quereda C, Lizan M, Martinez-Ferrer M. Colonization and infection with methicillin-resistant *Staphylococcus aureus*: associated factors and eradication. Infect Control Hosp Epidemiol 1996; 17:20–28.

9. Blot SI, Vandewoude KH, Hoste EA, Colardyn FA. Outcome and attributable mortality in critically ill patients with bacteremia involving methicillin-susceptible and methicillin-resistant *Staphylococcus aureus*. Arch Intern Med 2002; 162:2229–2235.

10. Chang FY, MacDonald BB, Peacock JE Jr, et al. A prospective multicenter study of *Staphylococcus aureus* bacteremia: incidence of endocarditis, risk factors for mortality, and clinical impact of methicillin resistance. Medicine (Baltimore) 2003; 82:322–332.

11. Combes A, Luyt CE, Fagon JY, et al. Impact of methicillin resistance on outcome of *Staphylococcus aureus* ventilator-associated pneumonia. Am J Respir Crit Care Med 2004; 170:786–792.

12. Cosgrove SE, Sakoulas G, Perencevich EN, Schwaber MJ, Karchmer AW, Carmeli Y. Comparison of mortality associated with methicillin-resistant and methicillin-susceptible *Staphylococcus aureus* bacteremia: a meta-analysis. Clin Infect Dis 2003; 36:53–59.

13. Fowler VG Jr, Olsen MK, Corey GR, et al. Clinical identifiers of complicated *Staphylococcus aureus* bacteremia. Arch Intern Med 2003; 163:2066–2072.

14. Gonzalez C, Rubio M, Romero-Vivas J, Gonzalez M, Picazo JJ. Bacteremic pneumonia due to *Staphylococcus aureus*: A comparison of disease caused by methicillin-resistant and methicillin-susceptible organisms. Clin Infect Dis 1999; 29:1171–1177.

15. Graffunder EM, Venezia RA. Risk factors associated with nosocomial methicillin-resistant *Staphylococcus aureus* (MRSA) infection including previous use of antimicrobials. J Antimicrob Chemother 2002; 49:999–1005.

16. Hershow RC, Khayr WF, Smith NL. A comparison of clinical virulence of nosocomially acquired methicillin-resistant and methicillin-sensitive *Staphylococcus aureus* infections in a university hospital. Infect Control Hosp Epidemiol 1992; 13:587–593.

17. Harbarth S, Rutschmann O, Sudre P, Pittet D. Impact of methicillin resistance on the outcome of patients with bacteremia caused by *Staphylococcus aureus*. Arch Intern Med 1998; 158:182–189.

18. Lodise TP Jr, McKinnon PS, Rybak M. Prediction model to identify patients with *Staphylococcus aureus* bacteremia at risk for methicillin resistance. Infect Control Hosp Epidemiol 2003; 24:655–661.

19. McHugh CG, Riley LW. Risk factors and costs associated with methicillin-resistant *Staphylococcus aureus* bloodstream infections. Infect Control Hosp Epidemiol 2004; 25:425–430.

20. Melzer M, Eykyn SJ, Gransden WR, Chinn S. Is methicillin-resistant *Staphylococcus aureus* more virulent than methicillin-susceptible *S. aureus*? A comparative cohort study of British patients with nosocomial infection and bacteremia. Clin Infect Dis 2003; 37:1453–1460.

21. Peacock JE Jr, Moorman DR, Wenzel RP, Mandell GL. Methicillin-resistant *Staphylococcus aureus*: microbiologic characteristics, antimicrobial susceptibilities, and assessment of virulence of an epidemic strain. J Infect Dis 1981; 144:575–582.

22. Romero-Vivas J, Rubio M, Fernandez C, Picazo JJ. Mortality associated with nosocomial bacteremia due to methicillin-resistant *Staphylococcus aureus*. Clin Infect Dis 1995; 21:1417–1423.

23. Soriano A, Martinez JA, Mensa J, et al. Pathogenic significance of methicillin resistance for patients with *Staphylococcus aureus* bacteremia. Clin Infect Dis 2000; 30:368–373.

24. Naimi TS, LeDell KH, Como-Sabetti K, et al. Comparison of community- and health care-associated methicillin-resistant *Staphylococcus aureus* infection. JAMA 2003; 290:2976–2984.

25. Rybak MJ, Pharm DK. Community-associated methicillin-resistant *Staphylococcus aureus*: a review. Pharmacotherapy 2005; 25:74–85.

26. Fridkin SK, Hageman JC, Morrison M, et al. Methicillin-resistant *Staphylococcus aureus* disease in three communities. N Engl J Med 2005; 352:1436–1444.

27. Ochoa TJ, Mohr J, Wanger A, Murphy JR, Heresi GP. Community-associated methicillin-resistant *Staphylococcus aureus* in pediatric patients. Emerg Infect Dis 2005; 11:966–968.

28. Harbarth S, Francois P, Shrenzel J, et al. Community-associated methicillin-resistant *Staphylococcus aureus*, Switzerland. Emerg Infect Dis 2005; 11: 962–965.

29. Moran GJ, Amii RN, Abrahamian FM, Talan DA. Methicillin-resistant *Staphylococcus aureus* in community-acquired skin infections. Emerg Infect Dis 2005; 11:928–930.

30. Mulvey MR, MacDougall L, Cholin B, Horsman G, Fidyk M, Woods S. Community-associated methicillin-resistant *Staphylococcus aureus*, Canada. Emerg Infect Dis 2005; 11:844–850.

31. Lee NE, Taylor MM, Bancroft E, et al. Risk factors for community-associated methicillin-resistant *Staphylococcus aureus* skin infections among HIV-positive men who have sex with men. Clin Infect Dis 2005; 40:1529–1534.

32. Nguyen DM, Mascola L, Brancoft E. Recurring methicillin-resistant *Staphylococcus aureus* infections in a football team. Emerg Infect Dis 2005; 11: 526–532.

33. Ribeiro A, Dias C, Silva-Carvalho MC, et al. First report of infection with community-acquired methicillin-resistant *Staphylococcus aureus* in South America. J Clin Microbiol 2005; 43:1985–1988.

34. Kazakova SV, Hageman JC, Matava M, et al. A clone of methicillin-resistant *Staphylococcus aureus* among professional football players. N Engl J Med 2005; 352:468–475.

35. Baillargeon J, Kelley MF, Leach CT, Baillargeon G, Pollock BH. Methicillin-resistant *Staphylococcus aureus* infection in the Texas prison system. Clin Infect Dis 2004; 38:e92–e95.

36. Pan ES, Diep BA, Carleton HA, et al. Increasing prevalence of methicillin-resistant *Staphylococcus aureus* infection in California jails. Clin Infect Dis 2003; 37:1384–1388.

37. Methicillin-resistant *Staphylococcus aureus* infections in correctional facilities—Georgia, California, and Texas, 2001–2003. MMWR Morb Mortal Wkly Rep 2003; 52:992–996.

38. Methicillin-resistant *Staphylococcus aureus* skin or soft tissue infections in a state prison—Mississippi, 2000. MMWR Morb Mortal Wkly Rep 2001; 50:919–922.

39. Shukla SK, Stemper ME, Ramaswamy SV, et al. Molecular characteristics of nosocomial and Native American community-associated methicillin-resistant *Staphylococcus aureus* clones from rural Wisconsin. J Clin Microbiol 2004; 42:3752–3757.

40. Whitener CJ, Park SY, Browne FA, et al. Vancomycin-resistant *Staphylococcus aureus* in the absence of vancomycin exposure. Clin Infect Dis 2004; 38:1049–1055.

41. *Staphylococcus aureus* resistant to vancomycin—United States, 2002. MMWR Morb Mortal Wkly Rep 2002; 51:565–567.

42. Vancomycin-resistant *Staphylococcus aureus*—Pennsylvania, 2002. MMWR Morb Mortal Wkly Rep 2002; 51:902.

43. Capitano B, Leshem OA, Nightingale CH, Nicolau DP. Cost effect of managing methicillin-resistant *Staphylococcus aureus* in a long-term care facility. J Am Geriatr Soc 2003; 51:10–16.

44. Chang FY, Peacock JE Jr, Musher DM, et al. *Staphylococcus aureus* bacteremia: recurrence and the impact of antibiotic treatment in a prospective multicenter study. Medicine (Baltimore) 2003; 82:333–339.

45. Cosgrove SE, Qi Y, Kaye KS, Harbarth S, Karchmer AW, Carmeli Y. The impact of methicillin resistance in *Staphylococcus aureus* bacteremia on patient outcomes: mortality, length of stay, and hospital charges. Infect Control Hosp Epidemiol 2005; 26:166–174.

46. Lodise TP, McKinnon PS, Swiderski L, Rybak MJ. Outcomes analysis of delayed antibiotic treatment for hospital-acquired *Staphylococcus aureus* bacteremia. Clin Infect Dis 2003; 36:1418–1423.

47. Rubin RJ, Harrington CA, Poon A, Dietrich K, Greene JA, Moiduddin A. The economic impact of *Staphylococcus aureus* infection in New York City hospitals. Emerg Infect Dis 1999; 5:9–17.

48. Whitby M, McLaws ML, Berry G. Risk of death from methicillin-resistant *Staphylococcus aureus* bacteraemia: a meta-analysis. Med J Aust 2001; 175:264–267.

49. Lodise TP, McKinnon PS. Clinical and economic impact of methicillin resistance in patients with *Staphylococcus aureus* bacteremia. Diagn Microbiol Infect Dis 2005; 52:113–122.

50. Wakefield DS, Helms CM, Massanari RM, Mori M, Pfaller M. Cost of nosocomial infection: relative contributions of laboratory, antibiotic, and per diem costs in serious *Staphylococcus aureus* infections. Am J Infect Control 1988; 16:185–192.

51. Engemann JJ, Carmeli Y, Cosgrove SE, et al. Adverse clinical and economic outcomes attributable to methicillin resistance among patients with *Staphylococcus aureus* surgical site infection. Clin Infect Dis 2003; 36:592–598.

52. Reed SD, Friedman JY, Engemann JJ, et al. Costs and outcomes among hemodialysis-dependent patients with methicillin-resistant or methicillin-susceptible *Staphylococcus aureus* bacteremia. Infect Control Hosp Epidemiol 2005; 26:175–183.

53. Cosgrove SE, Carmeli Y. The impact of antimicrobial resistance on health and economic outcomes. Clin Infect Dis 2003; 36:1433–1437.

54. Kim T, Oh PI, Simor AE. The economic impact of methicillin-resistant *Staphylococcus aureus* in Canadian hospitals. Infect Control Hosp Epidemiol 2001; 22:99–104.

55. Tice AD, Hoaglund PA, Nolet B, McKinnon PS, Mozaffari E. Cost perspectives for outpatient intravenous antimicrobial therapy. Pharmacotherapy 2002; 22:63S–70S.

56. Fowler VG Jr, Sakoulas G, McIntyre LM, et al. Persistent bacteremia due to methicillin-resistant *Staphylococcus aureus* infection is associated with agr dysfunction and low-level in vitro resistance to thrombin-induced platelet microbicidal protein. J Infect Dis 2004; 190:1140–1149.

57. Moise-Broder PA, Sakoulas G, Eliopoulos GM, Schentag JJ, Forrest A, Moellering RC Jr. Accessory gene regulator group II polymorphism in methicillin-resistant *Staphylococcus aureus* is predictive of failure of vancomycin therapy. Clin Infect Dis 2004; 38:1700–1705.

58. Sakoulas G, Eliopoulos GM, Moellering RC Jr, et al. *Staphylococcus aureus* accessory gene regulator (agr) group II: is there a relationship to the development of intermediate-level glycopeptide resistance? J Infect Dis 2003; 187:929–938.

59. Sakoulas G, Eliopoulos GM, Moellering RC Jr, et al. Accessory gene regulator (agr) locus in geographically diverse *Staphylococcus aureus* isolates with reduced susceptibility to vancomycin. Antimicrob Agents Chemother 2002; 46:1492–1502.

60. Sakoulas G, Moellering RC Jr, Eliopoulos GM. Adaptation of methicillin-resistant *Staphylococcus aureus* in the face of vancomycin therapy. Clin Infect Dis 2006; 42(suppl 1):S40–S50.

61. Ibrahim EH, Sherman G, Ward S, Fraser VJ, Kollef MH. The influence of inadequate antimicrobial treatment of bloodstream infections on patient outcomes in the ICU setting. Chest 2000; 118:146–155.

62. Leibovici L, Shraga I, Drucker M, Konigsberger H, Samra Z, Pitlik SD. The benefit of appropriate empirical antibiotic treatment in patients with bloodstream infection. J Intern Med 1998; 244:379–386.

63. Kollef MH, Ward S, Sherman G, et al. Inadequate treatment of nosocomial infections is associated with certain empiric antibiotic choices. Crit Care Med 2000; 28:3456–3464.

64. Sakoulas G, Moise-Broder PA, Schentag J, Forrest A, Moellering RC Jr, Eliopoulos GM. Relationship of MIC and bactericidal activity to efficacy of vancomycin for treatment of methicillin-resistant *Staphylococcus aureus* bacteremia. J Clin Microbiol 2004; 42:2398–2402.

65. Ariza J, Pujol M, Cabo J, et al. Vancomycin in surgical infections due to methicillin-resistant *Staphylococcus aureus* with heterogeneous resistance to vancomycin. Lancet 1999; 353:1587–1588.

66. Charles PG, Ward PB, Johnson PD, Howden BP, Grayson ML. Clinical features associated with bacteremia due to heterogeneous vancomycin-intermediate *Staphylococcus aureus*. Clin Infect Dis 2004; 38:448–451.

67. Cantoni L, Glauser MP, Bille J. Comparative efficacy of daptomycin, vancomycin, and cloxacillin for the treatment of *Staphylococcus aureus* endocarditis in rats and role of test conditions in this determination. Antimicrob Agents Chemother 1990; 34:2348–2353.

68. Levine DP, Fromm BS, Reddy BR. Slow response to vancomycin or vancomycin plus rifampin in methicillin-resistant *Staphylococcus aureus* endocarditis. Ann Intern Med 1991; 115:674–680.

69. Small PM, Chambers HF. Vancomycin for *Staphylococcus aureus* endocarditis in intravenous drug users. Antimicrob Agents Chemother 1990; 34:1227–1231.

70. Kollef MH, Rello J, Cammarata SK, Croos-Dabrera RV, Wunderink RG. Clinical cure and survival in Gram-positive ventilator-associated pneumonia: retrospective analysis of two double-blind studies comparing linezolid with vancomycin. Intensive Care Med 2004; 30:388–394.

71. Wunderink RG, Rello J, Cammarata SK, Croos-Dabrera RV, Kollef MH. Linezolid vs vancomycin: analysis of two double-blind studies of patients with methicillin-resistant *Staphylococcus aureus* nosocomial pneumonia. Chest 2003; 124:1789–1797.

72. Rubinstein E, Cammarata S, Oliphant T, Wunderink R. Linezolid (PNU-100766) versus vancomycin in the treatment of hospitalized patients with nosocomial pneumonia: a randomized, double-blind, multicenter study. Clin Infect Dis 2001; 32:402–412.

73. Cruciani M, Gatti G, Lazzarini L, et al. Penetration of vancomycin into human lung tissue. J Antimicrob Chemother 1996; 38:865–869.

74. Lamer C, de Beco V, Soler P, et al. Analysis of vancomycin entry into pulmonary lining fluid by bronchoalveolar lavage in critically ill patients. Antimicrob Agents Chemother 1993; 37:281–286.

75. Shorr AF, Susla GM, Kollef MH. Linezolid for treatment of ventilator-associated pneumonia: a cost-effective alternative to vancomycin. Crit Care Med 2004; 32:137–143.

76. Weigelt J, Itani K, Stevens D, Lau W, Dryden M, Knirsch C. Linezolid versus vancomycin in treatment of complicated skin and soft tissue infections. Antimicrob Agents Chemother 2005; 49:2260–2266.

77. Weigelt J, Kaafarani HM, Itani KM, Swanson RN. Linezolid eradicates MRSA better than vancomycin from surgical-site infections. Am J Surg 2004; 188:760–766.

78. Yaldo AZ, Sullivan JL, Li Z. Factors influencing physicians' decision to discharge hospitalized patients infected with methicillin-resistant *Staphylococcus aureus*. Am J Health Syst Pharm 2001; 58:1756–1759.

79. Parodi S, Rhew DC, Goetz MB. Early switch and early discharge opportunities in intravenous vancomycin treatment of suspected methicillin-resistant staphylococcal species infections. J Manag Care Pharm 2003; 9:317–326.

80. Li JZ, Willke RJ, Rittenhouse BE, Glick HA. Approaches to analysis of length of hospital stay related to antibiotic therapy in a randomized clinical trial: linezolid versus vancomycin for treatment of known or suspected methicillin-resistant *Staphylococcus* species infections. Pharmacotherapy 2002; 22:45S–54S.

81. Li JZ, Willke RJ, Rittenhouse BE, Rybak MJ. Effect of linezolid versus vancomycin on length of hospital stay in patients with complicated skin and soft tissue infections caused by known or suspected methicillin-resistant staphylococci: results from a randomized clinical trial. Surg Infect (Larchmt) 2003; 4:57–70.

82. Li Z, Willke RJ, Pinto LA, et al. Comparison of length of hospital stay for patients with known or suspected methicillin-resistant *Staphylococcus* species infections treated with linezolid or vancomycin: a randomized, multicenter trial. Pharmacotherapy 2001; 21:263–274.
83. McKinnon PS, Sorensen SV, Liu LZ, Itani KM. Impact of linezolid on economic outcomes and determinants of cost in a clinical trial evaluating patients with MRSA complicated skin and soft-tissue infections. Ann Pharmacother 2006; 40:1017–1023.
84. Itani KM, Weigelt J, Li JZ, Duttagupta S. Linezolid reduces length of stay and duration of intravenous treatment compared with vancomycin for complicated skin and soft tissue infections due to suspected or proven methicillin-resistant *Staphylococcus aureus* (MRSA). Int J Antimicrob Agents 2005; 26:442–448.

Index

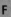

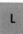

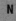
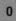

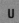
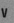